Ma Hochstetler

New FIRST PLACE Favorites

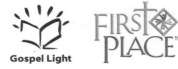

Gospel Light   FIRST PLACE™

Gospel Light is an evangelical Christian publisher dedicated to serving the local church. We believe God's vision for Gospel Light is to provide church leaders with biblical, user-friendly materials that will help them evangelize, disciple and minister to children, youth and families.

It is our prayer that this Gospel Light resource will help you discover biblical truth for your own life and help you minister to others. May God richly bless you.

For a free catalog of resources from Gospel Light, please contact your Christian supplier or contact us at 1-800-4-GOSPEL or www.gospellight.com.

PUBLISHING STAFF
William T. Greig, Chairman
Kyle Duncan, Publisher
Dr. Elmer L. Towns, Senior Consulting Publisher
Pam Weston, Managing Editor
Patti Pennington Virtue, Associate Editor
Hilary Young, Editorial Assistant
Jessie Minassian, Editorial Assistant
Bayard Taylor, M.Div., Senior Editor, Biblical and Theological Issues
Samantha A. Hsu, Cover Designer
Rosanne Moreland, Internal Designer
Lisa Lewis, Compiler

ISBN 0-8307-3231-4
© 2003 First Place
All rights reserved.
Printed in the U.S.A.

Any omission of credits is unintentional. The publisher requests documentation for future printings.

CAUTION
The information contained in this book is intended to be solely informational and educational. It is assumed that the First Place participant will consult a medical or health professional before beginning this or any other weight-loss or physical-fitness program.

Contents

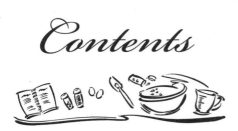

Preface 6

Helpful Information

Conversion Chart for Equivalent Imperial and Metric Measurements 7
Food Exchanges 10
First Place Grocery List 28

Recipes

APPETIZERS 31

BREADS 37
Biscuits and Rolls 38
Muffins 40
Miscellaneous 45

DESSERTS AND SWEETS 53
Beverages 54
Cakes and Pies 58
Frozen Treats 68
Gelatin Treats 71

Puddings 73
Miscellaneous 76

ENTRÉES 85
Beef and Venison 86
Fish and Seafood 99
Meatless Meals 103
Pork 110
Poultry 111

SIDE DISHES 131
Cooked Dishes 132
Salads, Slaws and Marinated Veggies 143

SOUPS 155

THIS 'N' THAT 163
Dips and Spreads 164
Gravy and Sauces 168
Salad Dressings 170
Miscellaneous 171

CONTRIBUTORS 173

INDEX 177

Preface

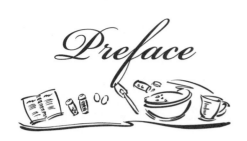

You are holding in your hand a great treasure. *New First Place Favorites* is a wonderful collection of recipes from faithful First Place members and leaders from all across our land. This is another valuable tool that can be used on your First Place journey.

I began my cooking career when I was eight years old. My mom worked outside the home, and I chose to take over many of the cooking responsibilities. As I spent hours watching my mom, dad, grandmother and a favorite aunt cook, I began to imitate their cooking skills. We did not own a recipe book, and I believe that is why I love getting my hands on a new recipe. I have always viewed a recipe as a suggestion. That concept has inspired many of the recipes in this book; many have taken an old family favorite, changed a few ingredients to make it fit the First Place healthy guidelines and, behold, a new creation for you and me to enjoy! Creating a new recipe is like a work of art to me, and I believe this collection is a First Place masterpiece.

First Place is a Bible-based weight-loss program that has been successfully used by over half a million people. First Place has proven that excess body fat can be lost without losing lean body mass. Members experience permanent weight loss by making daily healthy food choices and adopting an active lifestyle. The ultimate goal of each member is to attain balance in all areas of his or her life: physical, emotional, mental and spiritual. Members are encouraged to complete nine commitments to produce a positive transformation in each of these areas. Luke 2:52 states that "Jesus grew in wisdom and in stature, and in favor with God and men." First Place members learn how to use God's power in their daily lives.

Health officials agree that daily food choices can directly affect a person's health. Most of my cooking experience before First Place was with foods high in fat and sugar. First Place taught me the wonder of good-tasting dishes low in fat and low in sugar. Anyone who has an interest in a healthier lifestyle (or those experiencing health problems such as diabetes, heart disease, hypertension or cancer) will find many tasty and healthy choices in *New First Place Favorites*. May God bless you.

Kay Smith
First Place Associate National Director
www.firstplace.org

Conversion Chart for Equivalent Imperial and Metric Measurements

Liquid Measures

Fluid Ounces	U.S.	Imperial	Milliliters
	1 teaspoon	1 teaspoon	5
$\frac{1}{4}$	2 teaspoons	1 dessert spoon	7
$\frac{1}{2}$	1 tablespoon	1 tablespoon	15
1	2 tablespoons	2 tablespoons	28
2	$\frac{1}{4}$ cup	4 tablespoons	56
4	$\frac{1}{2}$ cup or $\frac{1}{4}$ pint		110
5		$\frac{1}{4}$ pint or 1 gill	140
6	$\frac{3}{4}$ cup		170
8	1 cup or $\frac{1}{2}$ pint		225
9			250 or $\frac{1}{4}$ liter
10	$1\frac{1}{4}$ cups	$\frac{1}{2}$ pint	280
12	$1\frac{1}{2}$ cups or $\frac{3}{4}$ pint		340
15		$\frac{3}{4}$ pint	420
16	2 cups or 1 pint		450
18	$2\frac{1}{4}$ cups		500 or $\frac{1}{2}$ liter
20	$2\frac{1}{2}$ cups	1 pint	560
24	3 cups or $1\frac{1}{2}$ pints		675
25		$1\frac{1}{4}$ pints	700
30	$3\frac{3}{4}$ cups	$1\frac{1}{2}$ pints	840
32	4 cups		900
36	$4\frac{1}{2}$ cups		1,000 or 1 liter
40	5 cups	2 pints or 1 quart	1,120
48	6 cups or 3 pints		1,350
50		$2\frac{1}{2}$ pints	1,400

Solid Measures

U.S. and Imperial Measures		Metric Measures	
Ounces	Pounds	Grams	Kilos
1		28	
2		56	
3½		100	
4	¼	112	
5		140	
6		168	
8	½	225	
9		250	¼
12	¾	340	
16	1	450	
18		500	½
20	1¼	560	
24		675	
27		750	¾
32	2	900	
36	2¼	1,000	1
40	2½	1,100	
48	3	1,350	
54		1,500	1½
64	4	1,800	
72	4½	2,000	2
80	5	2,250	2¼
100	6	2,800	2¾

Oven Temperature Equivalents

Fahrenheit	Celsius	Gas Mark	Description
225	110	¼	Cool
250	130	½	
275	140	1	Very Slow
300	150	2	
325	170	3	Slow
350	180	4	Moderate
375	190	5	
400	200	6	Moderately Hot
425	220	7	Fairly Hot
450	230	8	Hot
475	240	9	Very Hot
500	250	10	Extremely Hot

FOOD EXCHANGES

The food exchanges in this book are based on the American Dietetic Association, the United States Department of Agriculture and the American Diabetes Association dietary guidelines.

All recipe exchanges were determined using MasterCook software, a program that accesses a database containing over 6,000 food items prepared using the United States Department of Agriculture publications and information from food manufacturers. As with any nutritional program, MasterCook calculates the nutritional values of recipes based on ingredients. Nutrition may vary due to how the food is prepared and where the food comes from (i.e., soil content, season, ripeness, processing and method of preparation). For these reasons, please use the recipes as approximate guides.

The following daily exchange chart will help you to personalize your eating plan based on your nutritional needs and eating preferences. Choosing the lowest number of exchanges from each food group will give you fewer calories than listed in the chart. To stay within your desired calorie level, don't choose the higher number of exchanges for more than one food group. You can, however, choose the highest number of exchanges from the fruit and vegetable groups.

To determine your optimal daily calorie needs, consult with a physician and/or a registered dietician.

Daily Exchange Plans						
Levels	Bread/Starch	Vegetable	Fruit	Meat	Milk	Fat
1,200	5-6	3	2-3	4-5	2-3	3-4
1,400	6-7	3-4	3-4	5-6	2-3	3-4
1,500	7-8	3-4	3-4	5-6	2-3	3-4
1,600	8-9	3-4	3-4	6-7	2-3	3-4
1,800	10-11	3-4	3-4	6-7	2-3	4-5
2,000	11-12	4-5	4-5	6-7	2-3	5-6
2,200	12-13	4-5	4-5	7-8	2-3	6-7
2,400	13-14	4-5	4-5	8-9	2-3	7-8
2,600	14-15	5	5	9-10	2-3	7-8
2,800	15-16	5	5	9-10	2-3	9-10

Note: The food exchanges break down to approximately 50-55% carbohydrate, 15-20% protein and 25-30% fat.

ITEM	AMOUNT	EXCHANGES	
Alfalfa sprouts	1 c.	FREE	**A**
All-Bran cereal	½ c.	1 bread	
Almond butter	1 tsp.	1 fat	
Almonds, dry-roasted	6 whole	1 fat	
Animal crackers, low-fat, low-sugar	1 oz.	1 bread + ½ fat	
Apple	1 medium (4 oz.)	1 fruit	
Apple juice	½ c.	1 fruit	
Apples, dried	4 rings (¾ oz.)	1 fruit	
Applesauce, unsweetened	½ c.	1 fruit	
Apricots	4 medium	1 fruit	
Apricots, canned	½ c. (4 oz.)	1 fruit	
Apricots, dried	7 halves (¾ oz.)	1 fruit	
Artichoke, cooked	½ c.	1 vegetable	
Artichoke, raw	1 c.	1 vegetable	
Asparagus, cooked	½ c.	1 vegetable	
Asparagus, raw	1 c.	1 vegetable	
Avocado	⅛ medium	1 fat	
Bacon bits, imitation	^	FREE	**B**
Bacon grease	1 tsp.*	1 fat	
Bacon, pork	1 slice*	1 fat	
Bacon, turkey	2 slices	1 meat + ½ fat	
Bagel	½ (1 oz.)	1 bread	
Bamboo shoots, cooked	½ c.	1 vegetable	
Bamboo shoots, raw	1 c.	1 vegetable	
Banana	½ (3 oz.)	1 fruit	
Barbecue sauce	¼ c.	1 bread	
Barbecue sauce (as condiment)	^	FREE	

* Foods with this symbol are high in saturated fat and are not recommended.
^ Daily total for FREE foods with this symbol should not exceed 50 calories.

ITEM	AMOUNT	EXCHANGES
B Barley, cooked	⅓ c.	1 bread
Barley, dry	1½ tbsp.	1 bread
Bean sprouts, cooked	½ c.	1 vegetable
Bean sprouts, raw	1 c.	1 vegetable
Beans, baked	¼ c.	1 bread
Beans (green, Italian, wax), cooked	½ c.	1 vegetable
Beans (kidney, pinto, white), cooked	1 c.	2 breads + 1 lean meat
Beans (kidney, pinto, white), cooked	⅓ c.	1 bread
Beans, lima	½ c.	1 bread
Beans, refried	⅓ c.	1 bread + ½ fat
Beans, refried, fat-free	⅓ c.	1 bread
Beef, high-fat (prime cuts such as brisket, corned beef and ribs)	1 oz.	1 meat + 1 fat
Beef, lean (breakfast steak, filet mignon, flank steak, lean ground beef, London, broil, pot roast, sirloin, strip steak, tenderloin, top round)	1 oz.	1 meat
Beef, medium-fat (chuck roast, cubed steak, ground beef, Porterhouse steak, rib roast, rump roast, T-bone)	1 oz.	1 meat + ½ fat
Beets	½ c.	1 vegetable
Biscuit	1 medium (2½ in.)	1 bread + 1 fat
Blackberries	¾ c.	1 fruit
Blueberries	¾ c.	1 fruit
Bok choy	1 c.	FREE
Bologna	1 oz.	1 meat + 1 fat
Bouillon	^	FREE
Boysenberries	¾ c.	1 fruit
Bran cereal, concentrated	⅓ c.	1 bread
Bran cereal, flaked	½ c.	1 bread
Bran, raw, unprocessed	½ c.	1 bread

* Foods with this symbol are high in saturated fat and are not recommended.
^ Daily total for FREE foods with this symbol should not exceed 50 calories.

ITEM	AMOUNT	EXCHANGES	
Bratwurst	1 oz.	1 meat + 1 fat	**B**
Bread crumbs, dried	2 tbsp.	1 bread	
Bread, diet (40 calories per slice)	2 slices	1 bread	
Bread, pumpernickel	1 slice (1 oz.)	1 bread	
Bread, rye	1 slice (1 oz.)	1 bread	
Bread, whole-wheat, white, French, Italian	1 slice (1 oz.)	1 bread	
Breadsticks, crisp	2 4x1½-in.	1 bread	
Broccoli, cooked	½ c.	1 vegetable	
Broccoli, raw	1 c.	1 vegetable	
Broth	^	FREE	
Bulgur, cooked	½ c.	1 bread	
Bun, hamburger or hot dog	½ (1 oz.)	1 bread	
Butter	1 tsp.*	1 fat	
Butter flavoring, powdered	^	FREE	
Butter, reduced-fat	1 tbsp.*	1 fat	
Buttermilk, fat-free	1 c.	1 milk	
Cabbage, Chinese	1 c.	FREE	**C**
Cabbage, cooked	½ c.	1 vegetable	
Cabbage, raw	1 c.	FREE	
Canadian bacon	1 oz.	1 meat	
Candies, sugar-free	^	FREE	
Cantaloupe	⅓ melon (7 oz.) or 1 c. cubed	1 fruit	
Carambola (starfruit)	3 (7½ oz.)	1 fruit	
Carbonated sugar-free soda	^	FREE	
Carbonated water	^	FREE	
Carrot juice	½ c.	1 vegetable	

* Foods with this symbol are high in saturated fat and are not recommended.
^ Daily total for FREE foods with this symbol should not exceed 50 calories.

ITEM	AMOUNT	EXCHANGES
Cashews, dry-roasted	1 tbsp.	1 fat
Catsup	¼ c.	1 bread
Catsup (as condiment)	^	FREE
Celery	1 c.	FREE
Cereal, 100% bran	⅓ c.	1 bread
Cereal, cooked	½ c.	1 bread
Cereal, ready-to-eat, unsweetened	¾ c.	1 bread
Cheerios	¾ c.	1 bread
Cheese	2 oz.	1 milk
Cheese (all regular cheeses such as American, blue, cheddar, Colby, Monterey, Jack and Swiss)	1 oz.	1 meat + 1 fat
Cheese, fat-free	1 oz.	1 meat
Cheese (light, skim or part-skim milk cheeses)	1 oz.	1 meat + ½ fat
Cheese, Parmesan, grated	2 tbsp.	1 meat
Cheese spread	1 tbsp.*	1 fat
Cherries, raw	12 large (3½ oz.)	1 fruit
Cherries, canned	½ c.	1 fruit
Chewing gum, sugar-free	^	FREE
Chicken, baked	1 oz.	1 meat + 1 fat
Chicken fat	1 tsp.*	1 fat
Chicken, fried	1 oz.	1 meat + 1 fat
Chicken noodle soup, canned	1 c.	½ bread + ½ fat
Chili sauce	¼ c.	1 bread
Chili sauce (as condiment)	^	FREE
Chips, corn	1 oz.	1 bread + 2 fats
Chips, potato	1 oz.	1 bread + 2 fats
Chips, tortilla	5	1 bread
Chitterlings	½ oz.*	1 fat
Chocolate, baking	1 oz.	1 bread + 2 fats

* Foods with this symbol are high in saturated fat and are not recommended.
^ Daily total for FREE foods with this symbol should not exceed 50 calories.

ITEM	AMOUNT	EXCHANGES
Chocolate, unsweetened	1 oz.*	1 bread + 2 fats
Chocolate-milk mix, sugar-free	^	FREE
Chow mein noodles	½ c.	1 bread + 1 fat
Cilantro	1 c.	FREE
Club soda	^	FREE
Cocktail sauce	^	FREE
Cocoa	5 tbsp.	1 bread
Cocoa powder, unsweetened	^	FREE
Coconut, shredded	2 tbsp.*	1 fat
Coffee	^	FREE
Coffee whitener, liquid	2 tbsp.*	1 fat
Coffee whitener, nondairy	^	FREE
Coffee whitener, powder	4 tsp.*	1 fat
Cooking spray	^	FREE
Corn	½ c.	1 bread
Cornbread	1 2-in. cube (2 oz.)	1 bread + 1 fat
Cornflakes	¾ c.	1 bread
Cornish game hen	1 oz.	1 meat
Cornmeal	2½ tbsp.	1 bread
Corn-on-the-cob	1 6-in. ear	1 bread
Cornstarch	2 tbsp.	1 bread
Cottage cheese	¼ c.	1 meat
Cottage cheese	½ c.	1 milk
Couscous, cooked	⅓ c.	1 bread
Crab apples	¾ c. (2¾ oz.)	1 fruit
Crackers, round butter-type	6	1 bread + 1 fat
Crackers, saltine	6	1 bread
Cranberry juice	⅓ c.	1 fruit
Cream cheese	1 tbsp.*	1 fat

* Foods with this symbol are high in saturated fat and are not recommended.
^ Daily total for FREE foods with this symbol should not exceed 50 calories.

C

	ITEM	AMOUNT	EXCHANGES
C	Cream cheese, fat-free	2 oz.	1 meat
	Cream cheese, light	2 tbsp.*	1 fat
	Cream, half-and-half	2 tbsp.*	1 fat
	Cream of broccoli soup, canned	½ c.	1 bread
	Cream of celery soup, canned	½ c.	1 bread
	Cream of chicken soup, canned	½ c.	1 bread + 1 fat
	Cream of mushroom soup, canned	½ c.	½ bread + ½ fat
	Cress, garden	1 c.	FREE
	Croissant	1 small	1 bread + 2 fats
	Croutons, low-fat	1 c.	1 bread
	Cucumber	1 c.	FREE
D	Dates, dried	2½ medium	1 fruit
	Dewberries	¾ c. (3 oz.)	1 fruit
	Drink mixes, sugar-free	^	FREE
	Dry nonfat milk	¼ c.	1 milk
	Duck	1 oz.	1 meat + ½ fat
E	Egg	1	1 meat + ½ fat
	Egg substitutes	¼ c.	1 meat
	Egg whites	3	1 meat
	Eggplant, cooked	½ c.	1 vegetable
	Eggplant, raw	1 c.	1 vegetable
	Enchilada sauce	^	FREE
	Endive	1 c.	FREE
	English muffin	½	1 bread
	Escarole	1 c.	FREE

* Foods with this symbol are high in saturated fat and are not recommended.
^ Daily total for FREE foods with this symbol should not exceed 50 calories.

FOOD EXCHANGES

ITEM	AMOUNT	EXCHANGES	
Evaporated nonfat milk	½ c.	1 milk	**E**
Evaporated whole milk	½ c.	1 milk + 2 fats	
Fiber One cereal	⅔ c.	1 bread	**F**
Figs, dried	1½	1 fruit	
Figs	2 2-in.	1 fruit	
Fish (canned tuna in oil and canned salmon)	¼ c.	1 meat + ½ fat	
Fish (catfish, haddock, halibut, herring, orange roughy, trout, salmon or tuna in water), baked	1 oz.	1 meat	
Fish, fried	1 oz.	1 meat + 1 fat	
Flour, soybean	½ c.	1 bread + 2 meats + 1 fat	
Flour, white or whole-wheat	1 c.	5 breads	
Frankfurter, low-fat	1 oz.	1 meat	
Frankfurter (up to 5 grams fat/oz.)	1 oz.	1 meat + ½ fat	
Frankfurter (up to 8 grams of fat/oz.)	1 oz.	1 meat + 1 fat	
French fries (2 to 3½ in. long)	10 fries	1 bread + 1 fat	
Fruit cocktail, canned	½ c.	1 fruit	
Fruit spreads, sugar-free	^	FREE	
Game (venison, rabbit)	1 oz.	1 meat	**G**
Gelatin, sugar-free	^	FREE	
Goose	1 oz.	1 meat + ½ fat	
Gooseberries	1 c. (5 oz.)	1 fruit	
Graham crackers	3 2-in. squares	1 bread	
Grape juice	⅓ c.	1 fruit	
Grapefruit	½ grapefruit	1 fruit	
Grapefruit juice	½ c.	1 fruit	

* Foods with this symbol are high in saturated fat and are not recommended.
^ Daily total for FREE foods with this symbol should not exceed 50 calories.

	ITEM	AMOUNT	EXCHANGES
G	Grapefruit, segments	¾ c.	1 fruit
	Grape-Nuts flakes	½ c.	1 bread
	Grape-Nuts nuggets	3 tbsp.	1 bread
	Grapes	17 small	1 fruit
	Gravy, home-style	¼ c.*	1 fat
	Gravy, packaged	½ c.*	1 fat
	Green onion	1 c.	FREE
	Grits, cooked	½ c.	1 bread
	Ground pork	1 oz.	1 meat + 1 fat
	Ground turkey	1 oz.	1 meat + ½ fat
H	Ham	1 oz.	1 meat
	Heart	1 oz.	1 meat + ½ fat
	Hearts of palm, cooked	½ c.	1 vegetable
	Hearts of palm, raw	1 c.	1 vegetable
	Hominy	½ c.	1 bread
	Honeydew melon, cubed	1 c.	1 fruit
	Honeydew melon, sliced	⅛ melon	1 fruit
	Horseradish	^	FREE
	Hot chocolate, sugar-free	1 packet	½ milk
	Hot peppers	1 c.	FREE
	Hummus	¼ c.	1 bread + 1 fat
I	Ice cream, sugar-free, fat-free	3 oz.	1 bread
	Ice-cream bar, sugar-free	^	FREE
	Iced tea, sugar-free	^	FREE

* Foods with this symbol are high in saturated fat and are not recommended.
^ Daily total for FREE foods with this symbol should not exceed 50 calories.

ITEM	AMOUNT	EXCHANGES	
Jicama, cooked	½ c.	1 vegetable	**J**
Jicama, raw	1 c.	1 vegetable	
Kale, cooked	½ c.	1 vegetable	**K**
Kale, raw	1 c.	1 vegetable	
Kasha, cooked	½ c.	1 bread	
Kidney	1 oz.	1 meat + ½ fat	
Kiwi	1 large (3 ¼ oz.)	1 fruit	
Knockwurst	1 oz.	1 meat + 1 fat	
Kohlrabi, cooked	½ c.	1 vegetable	
Kohlrabi, raw	1 c.	1 vegetable	
Lactaid	1 c.	1 milk	**L**
Lamb (chops, leg and roast)	1 oz.	1 meat + ½ fat	
Lamb, ground	1 oz.	1 meat + 1 fat	
Lard	1 tsp.*	1 fat	
Leeks, cooked	½ c.	1 vegetable	
Leeks, raw	½ c.	1 vegetable	
Lemon juice	1 c.	1 fruit	
Lemon juice (as seasoning)	^	FREE	
Lentils	1 c.	2 breads + 1 lean meat	
Lentils (as a side)	⅓ c.	1 bread	
Lettuce	1 c.	FREE	
Lime juice	1 c.	1 fruit	
Lime juice (as seasoning)	^	FREE	
Liver	1 oz.	1 meat + ½ fat	
Luncheon meat, fat-free	1 oz.	1 meat	

* Foods with this symbol are high in saturated fat and are not recommended.
^ Daily total for FREE foods with this symbol should not exceed 50 calories.

ITEM	AMOUNT	EXCHANGES
L		
Luncheon meat, high-fat (bologna, salami, pimiento loaf)	1 oz.	1 meat + 1 fat
Luncheon meat, lean (up to 5 grams of fat)	1 oz.	1 meat + ½ fat
M		
Malt (dry)	1 tbsp.	1 bread
Mandarin oranges, canned in own juice	¾ c.	1 fruit
Mango	½ mango (3 oz.)	1 fruit
Margarine	1 tsp.	1 fat
Margarine, light	1 tbsp.	1 fat
Matzo	¾ oz.	1 bread
Mayonnaise	1 tsp.	1 fat
Mayonnaise, fat-free	^	FREE
Mayonnaise, light	1 tbsp.	1 fat
Meat fat	1 tsp.*	1 fat
Melba toast	5 slices	1 bread
Milk, 1½% or 2%	1 c.	1 milk + 1 fat
Milk, 1%	1 c.	1 milk + ½ fat
Milk, nonfat or ½%	1 c.	1 milk
Milk, whole	1 c.	1 milk + 2 fats
Millet, cooked	¼ c.	1 bread
Miso	½ c.	1 bread + 2 meats + 1 fat
Muffin, plain	1 small	1 bread + 1 fat
Mulberries	1 c. (5 oz.)	1 fruit
Mushrooms, cooked	½ c.	1 vegetable
Mushrooms, raw	1 c.	FREE
Mustard	^	FREE

* Foods with this symbol are high in saturated fat and are not recommended.
^ Daily total for FREE foods with this symbol should not exceed 50 calories.

ITEM	AMOUNT	EXCHANGES
Nectarine	1 medium (5 oz.)	1 fruit
Nuts, chopped (almonds, pecans, walnuts)	1 tbsp.	1 fat
Oil (corn, cottonseed, olive, peanut, safflower, soybean and sunflower)	1 tsp.	1 fat
Okra	1 c.	1 vegetable
Onion, cooked	½ c.	1 vegetable
Onion, raw	1 c.	1 vegetable
Orange	1 medium (6½ oz.)	1 fruit
Orange juice	½ c.	1 fruit
Orange juice concentrate	2 tbsp. (1 oz.)	1 fruit
Oyster crackers	24	1 bread
Pancake	2 4-in.	1 bread + 1 fat
Papaya	1 c. (8 oz.)	1 fruit
Parsley	1 c.	FREE
Passion fruit	4 4 oz.	1 fruit
Pasta, cooked	½ c.	1 bread
Pea pods	½ c.	1 vegetable
Peaches	1 peach or ¾ c.	1 fruit
Peaches, canned	½ c. or 2 halves	1 fruit
Peanut butter, low-fat or regular	1 tsp.	1 fat
Peanut butter, low-fat or regular	1 tbsp.	1 meat + 1 fat
Peanuts	20 small or 10 large	1 fat
Pear, canned	½ c. or 2 halves	1 fruit
Pear with skin	½ large or 1 small	1 fruit
Peas (black-eyed, split), cooked (as a side)	⅓ c.	1 bread
Peas (black-eyed, split), cooked	1 c.	2 bread + 1 lean meat

N

O

P

* Foods with this symbol are high in saturated fat and are not recommended.
^ Daily total for FREE foods with this symbol should not exceed 50 calories.

ITEM	AMOUNT	EXCHANGES
P Peas, green	½ c.	1 bread
Pecans	2 large	1 fat
Peppers (all varieties)	^	FREE
Persimmon	2 medium	1 fruit
Picante sauce	^	FREE
Pickle relish	^	FREE
Pickles, unsweetened	^	FREE
Pimiento	3 oz.	1 vegetable
Pimiento loaf	1 oz.	1 meat + 1 fat
Pineapple, canned in own juice	⅓ c.	1 fruit
Pineapple	¾ c.	1 fruit
Pineapple juice	½ c.	1 fruit
Pine nuts	1 tbsp.	1 fat
Pita	½ 6-in.	1 bread
Plantain	½ c.	1 bread
Plums	2 small (5 oz.)	1 fruit
Pomegranate	½ medium	1 fruit
Popcorn, air-popped (no fat added)	3 c.	1 bread
Pork chops	1 oz.	1 meat + ½ fat
Pork, high-fat (ground pork, pork sausage, spareribs)	1 oz.	1 meat + 1 fat
Pork, lean (boiled, canned, cured or fresh ham, Canadian bacon, tenderloin)	1 oz.	1 meat
Pork, medium-fat (Boston butts, chops, cutlets, loin roast)	1 oz.	1 meat + ½ fat
Pork sausage	1 oz.	1 meat + 1 fat
Potato, baked	1 small	1 bread
Potato, mashed	½ c.	1 bread
Potato, sweet, plain	⅓ c.	1 bread

* Foods with this symbol are high in saturated fat and are not recommended.
^ Daily total for FREE foods with this symbol should not exceed 50 calories.

ITEM	AMOUNT	EXCHANGES	
Poultry (chicken with skin, domestic duck or goose ground turkey)	1 oz.	1 meat + ½ fat	**P**
Poultry (Cornish game hen, skinless chicken, turkey)	1 oz.	1 meat	
Pretzels	¾ oz.	1 bread	
Prune juice	⅓ c.	1 fruit	
Prunes, dried	3 medium (1 oz.)	1 fruit	
Pudding, sugar-free, prepared with fat-free milk	½ c.	½ milk + ½ bread	
Puffed cereal (rice, wheat)	1½ c.	1 bread	
Pumpkin, canned	¾ c.	1 bread	
Pumpkin, home-cooked	¾ c.	½ bread	
Pumpkin seeds	2 tsp.	1 fat	
Radishes	1 c.	FREE	**R**
Raisin Bran cereal	½ c.	1 bread	
Raisin bread (unfrosted)	1 slice (1 oz.)	1 bread	
Raisins	2 tbsp. (¼ oz.)	1 fruit	
Raspberries	1 c.	1 fruit	
Rhubarb, diced	2 c.	1 fruit	
Rice (brown), cooked	½ c.	1 bread	
Rice cakes	2 regular or 6 mini	1 bread	
Rice Krispies	¾ c.	1 bread	
Rice (white), cooked	⅓ c.	1 bread	
Rice (wild), cooked	½ c.	1 bread	
Ricotta cheese	¼ c.	1 meat + ½ fat	
Roll, butter-style	1 small (1 oz.)	1 bread + 1 fat	
Roll, dinner	1 small (1 oz.)	1 bread	
Romaine lettuce	1 c.	FREE	
Rutabaga	1 c.	1 vegetable	
Rye Krisp	4 2x3½-in.	1 bread	

* Foods with this symbol are high in saturated fat and are not recommended.
^ Daily total for FREE foods with this symbol should not exceed 50 calories.

ITEM	AMOUNT	EXCHANGES
S		
Salad dressing, fat-free	^	FREE
Salad dressing, light	1 tbsp.	1 fat
Salad dressing, regular	1 tsp.	1 fat
Salami	1 oz.	1 meat +1 fat
Salsa	^	FREE
Salt pork	¼ oz.*	1 fat
Salt, seasoned	^	FREE
Sauerkraut	1 c.	1 vegetable
Sausage (Italian, pork, etc.)	1 oz.	1 meat +1 fat
Shake, nutritional sugar-free (e.g., Alba Shake)	1 packet	1 milk
Shallots	4 tbsp.	1 vegetable
Shellfish (clams, crab, lobster, scallops, shrimp)	2 oz.	1 meat
Shortening	1 tsp.*	1 fat
Shredded wheat cereal	½ c.	1 bread
Shrimp, fried	2 oz.	1 meat + 1 fat
Snow peas	½ c.	1 vegetable
Soup, chicken noodle, canned	1 c.	½ bread + ½ fat
Soup, cream of broccoli, canned	½ c.	1 bread
Soup, cream of celery, canned	½ c.	1 bread
Soup, cream of chicken, canned	½ c.	1 bread + 1 fat
Soup, cream of mushroom, canned	½ c.	½ bread+ 1 fat
Soup, vegetable beef, canned	1 c.	1 bread
Soup, vegetable, canned	1 c.	1 bread
Sour cream	2 tbsp.*	1 fat
Sour cream, fat-free	^	FREE
Sour cream, light	3 tbsp.*	1 fat
Soy sauce	^	FREE
Spareribs	1 oz.	1 meat + 1 fat

* Foods with this symbol are high in saturated fat and are not recommended.
^ Daily total for FREE foods with this symbol should not exceed 50 calories.

ITEM	AMOUNT	EXCHANGES	
Spinach, cooked	½ c.	1 vegetable	**S**
Spinach, raw	1 c.	FREE	
Squash, cooked	¾ c.	1 bread	
Steak sauce	^	FREE	
Strawberries	1¼ c.	1 fruit	
Strawberries, frozen	1 c.	1 fruit	
Stuffing, bread, prepared	¼ c.	1 bread + 1 fat	
Sugar substitutes (all)	^	FREE	
Sunflower seeds, shelled	1 tbsp.	1 fat	
Sweetbreads (high in cholesterol)	1 oz.	1 meat + ½ fat	
Syrup, sugar-free	^	FREE	
Tabasco sauce	^	FREE	**T**
Tabouli	2 tbsp.	1 bread + 1 fat	
Taco sauce	^	FREE	
Taco shell	1 6-in.	1 bread + 1 fat	
Tangelo	1 medium	1 fruit	
Tangerines	2 small (8 oz.)	1 fruit	
Tapioca	2 tbsp.	1 bread	
Tea (all types), unsweetened	^	FREE	
Tempeh	½ c.	1 bread + 2 meats + 1 fat	
Teriyaki sauce	^	FREE	
Tofu	4 oz.	1 meat + ½ fat	
Tomato	1 large	1 vegetable	
Tomato juice	½ c.	1 vegetable	
Tomato paste	6 tbsp.	1 bread	
Tomato sauce	1 c.	1 bread	
Tomato sauce (as condiment)	^	FREE	

* Foods with this symbol are high in saturated fat and are not recommended.
^ Daily total for FREE foods with this symbol should not exceed 50 calories.

	ITEM	AMOUNT	EXCHANGES
T	Tonic water	^	FREE
	Tortilla chips, baked	1 oz.	1 bread + 1 fat
	Tortilla, corn	1 6-in.	1 bread
	Tortilla, flour	1 6-in.	1 bread + 1 fat
	Tuna, canned in oil	¼ c.	1 meat + ½ fat
	Tuna, canned in water	¼ c.	1 meat
	Turkey	1 oz.	1 meat
	Turkey bacon	2 slices	1 meat + ½ fat
	Turnips, cooked	½ c.	1 vegetable
	Turnips, raw	1 c.	1 vegetable
V	Vanilla wafers, low-fat	8	1 bread + ½ fat
	Veal, cutlet (ground or cubed, not breaded)	1 oz.	1 meat + ½ fat
	Veal, lean (all are lean except cutlets)	1 oz.	1 meat
	Vegetable beef soup, canned	1 c.	1 bread
	Vegetable juice	½ c.	1 vegetable
	Vegetable soup, canned	1 c.	1 bread
	Vinegar (all types)	^	FREE
W	Waffle	1 5x5x½-in.	1 bread + 1 fat
	Walnuts	2 whole	1 fat
	Water chestnuts	½ c.	1 vegetable
	Watercress	1 c.	FREE
	Watermelon, cubed	1¼ c.	1 fruit
	Wheat germ, raw	3 tbsp.	1 bread
	Wheat germ, toasted	¼ c.	1 bread + 1 lean meat
	Wheaties	¾ c.	1 bread

* Foods with this symbol are high in saturated fat and are not recommended.
^ Daily total for FREE foods with this symbol should not exceed 50 calories.

ITEM	AMOUNT	EXCHANGES	
Whipped topping	3 tbsp.*	1 fat	**W**
Whipped topping, fat-free	^	FREE	
Whipping cream	1 tbsp.*	1 fat	
Worcestershire sauce	^	FREE	
Yam, sweet potato, plain	⅓ c.	1 bread	**Y**
Yogurt, fat-free and sugar-free	8 oz.	1 milk	
Yogurt, frozen, nonfat	3 oz.	1 bread	
Yogurt, low-fat sugar-free	8 oz.	1 milk + 1 fat	
Yogurt, plain sugar-free	8 oz.	1 milk + 2 fats	
Zucchini, cooked	½ c.	1 vegetable	**Z**
Zucchini, raw	1 c.	FREE	

* Foods with this symbol are high in saturated fat and are not recommended.
^ Daily total for FREE foods with this symbol should not exceed 50 calories.

FIRST PLACE GROCERY LIST

Use this list to get you started, and make copies so that you will have a list for each week.

BAKING GOODS

- [ ] ____ Baking powder
- [ ] ____ Baking soda
- [ ] ____ Cocoa
- [ ] ____ Cornstarch
- [ ] ____ Herbs, dried
- [ ] ____ Nuts
- [ ] ____ Pepper
- [ ] ____ Raisins
- [ ] ____ Salt
- [ ] ____ Spices
- [ ] ____ Vanilla
- [ ] _____
- [ ] _____

BEVERAGES

- [ ] ____ Cocoa
- [ ] ____ Coffee
- [ ] ____ Fruit juice, 100%
- [ ] ____ Mineral water
- [ ] ____ Soft drinks, diet
- [ ] ____ Tea
- [ ] _____
- [ ] _____

BREADS

- [ ] ____ Bagels
- [ ] ____ Breads
- [ ] ____ Buns
- [ ] ____ English muffins
- [ ] ____ Rolls
- [ ] _____
- [ ] _____
- [ ] _____
- [ ] _____

CANNED GOODS

- [ ] ____ Applesauce
- [ ] ____ Beans
- [ ] ____ Chili
- [ ] ____ Fruit
- [ ] ____ Mushrooms
- [ ] ____ Soup
- [ ] ____ Spaghetti sauce
- [ ] ____ Tomato paste
- [ ] ____ Tomato sauce
- [ ] ____ Tomatoes, stewed
- [ ] ____ Tuna/salmon
- [ ] ____ Vegetables
- [ ] _____
- [ ] _____
- [ ] _____
- [ ] _____

CONDIMENTS

- [ ] ____ All-fruit/jam/jelly
- [ ] ____ Honey
- [ ] ____ Ketchup
- [ ] ____ Mayonnaise, low-fat
- [ ] ____ Mustard
- [ ] ____ Oil, olive
- [ ] ____ Oil, vegetable
- [ ] ____ Olives
- [ ] ____ Peanut butter
- [ ] ____ Pickles
- [ ] ____ Relish
- [ ] ____ Salad dressings
- [ ] ____ Salsa
- [ ] ____ Soy sauce
- [ ] ____ Syrup, diet
- [ ] ____ Vinegar

DAIRY

- [ ] ____ Butter, reduced-fat
- [ ] ____ Cheese, other
- [ ] ____ Cheese, parmesan
- [ ] ____ Cottage cheese
- [ ] ____ Cream cheese
- [ ] ____ Eggs/egg sub.
- [ ] ____ Milk, nonfat/1%
- [ ] ____ Margarine, reduced-calorie
- [ ] ____ Margarine, reduced-fat
- [ ] ____ Sour Cream, low-fat
- [ ] ____ Yogurt, 90-calorie
- [ ] _____
- [ ] _____
- [ ] _____
- [ ] _____

DRY GOODS

- [ ] _____ Beans/peas/lentils
- [ ] _____ Bread crumbs
- [ ] _____ Cereals
- [ ] _____ Chips, tortilla
- [ ] _____ Cornmeal
- [ ] _____ Crackers
- [ ] _____ Flour
- [ ] _____ Oatmeal
- [ ] _____ Pancake mix
- [ ] _____ Pasta/noodles
- [ ] _____ Pudding, sugar-free
- [ ] _____ Rice
- [ ] _____ Sugar/sugar sub.
- [ ] _____ _____
- [ ] _____ _____
- [ ] _____ _____
- [ ] _____ _____
- [ ] _____ _____

FROZEN FOODS

- [ ] _____ Dinners, frozen
- [ ] _____ Ice cream, light
- [ ] _____ Vegetables
- [ ] _____ Waffles, frozen
- [ ] _____ Whipped topping, light
- [ ] _____ Yogurt, light
- [ ] _____ _____
- [ ] _____ _____
- [ ] _____ _____
- [ ] _____ _____
- [ ] _____ _____

FRUIT

- [ ] _____ Apples
- [ ] _____ Bananas
- [ ] _____ Berries
- [ ] _____ Grapefruit
- [ ] _____ Grapes
- [ ] _____ Lemons

- [ ] _____ Limes
- [ ] _____ Melons
- [ ] _____ Oranges
- [ ] _____ Pears
- [ ] _____ _____
- [ ] _____ _____
- [ ] _____ _____
- [ ] _____ _____
- [ ] _____ _____

MEAT, FISH, POULTRY

- [ ] _____ Bacon, turkey
- [ ] _____ Beef, ground, lean
- [ ] _____ Beef, lean
- [ ] _____ Chicken
- [ ] _____ Deli Meat
- [ ] _____ Fish
- [ ] _____ Ham, lean
- [ ] _____ Hot dogs, low-fat
- [ ] _____ Pork tenderloin
- [ ] _____ Sausage, low-fat
- [ ] _____ Shellfish
- [ ] _____ Turkey
- [ ] _____ _____
- [ ] _____ _____
- [ ] _____ _____
- [ ] _____ _____
- [ ] _____ _____

VEGETABLES

- [ ] _____ Broccoli
- [ ] _____ Cabbage
- [ ] _____ Carrots
- [ ] _____ Cauliflower
- [ ] _____ Celery
- [ ] _____ Cucumbers
- [ ] _____ Garlic
- [ ] _____ Lettuce
- [ ] _____ Mushrooms

- [ ] _____ Onions
- [ ] _____ Peppers
- [ ] _____ Potatoes
- [ ] _____ Radishes
- [ ] _____ Spinach
- [ ] _____ Tomatoes
- [ ] _____ _____
- [ ] _____ _____
- [ ] _____ _____
- [ ] _____ _____
- [ ] _____ _____
- [ ] _____ _____
- [ ] _____ _____

MISCELLANEOUS

- [ ] _____ _____
- [ ] _____ _____
- [ ] _____ _____
- [ ] _____ _____
- [ ] _____ _____
- [ ] _____ _____
- [ ] _____ _____
- [ ] _____ _____
- [ ] _____ _____
- [ ] _____ _____
- [ ] _____ _____
- [ ] _____ _____
- [ ] _____ _____
- [ ] _____ _____
- [ ] _____ _____
- [ ] _____ _____

APPETIZERS

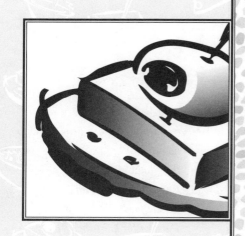

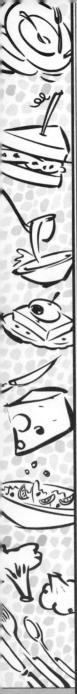

Appetizers

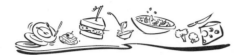

10 hard-boiled eggs
¾ c. mashed potatoes, prepared with
    nonfat milk
1 tbsp. light mayonnaise
1 tsp. prepared mustard
   Yellow food coloring (optional)
   Paprika for garnish

NO-YOLK DEVILED EGGS

Contributed by Evelyn Bailey, New Orleans, Louisiana

Slice eggs in half lengthwise; remove yolks and refrigerate for another use. Set whites aside. In small bowl, combine mashed potatoes, mayonnaise, mustard and 2 drops food coloring, if desired; mix well and refill egg whites with mixture. Sprinkle with paprika; refrigerate until ready to serve. Serves 10.
Exchanges: ⅓ **meat**

PARTY SANDWICH

Contributed by Carol Moore, Meridian, Mississippi

Preheat oven to 400° F. Slice off top of bread loaf; set top aside. Hollow out inside of loaf and save crumbs for another use. In small bowl, combine mayonnaise, Italian seasoning and pepper. Use half of mayonnaise mixture to thinly coat inside of bread shell; set aside. In small skillet, use olive oil to sauté onion, peppers and celery until tender; remove from heat and set aside. Layer ½ each of ham, vegetables and cheese inside bread shell; top with remaining mayonnaise mixture; repeat with remaining ham, vegetables and cheese. Replace bread top; wrap in heavy-duty foil. Bake 30 minutes; remove and slice to serve. Serves 4.
Exchanges: 3 breads, 2 lean meats, 1 vegetable, 1 fat

PINEAPPLE CHEESE BALL

Contributed by Janet Bayless, Clinton, Tennessee

In small bowl, use fork to blend cream cheese until smooth. Gradually stir in pineapple, ½ of pecans, green pepper, onion and salt. Mix well; shape into a ball with hands and set aside. Spread remaining pecans on wax paper; roll cheese ball over pecans until ball is covered (continue rolling until all pecans are used). Wrap cheese ball in plastic wrap and refrigerate overnight. Serves 16.
Exchanges: ½ meat, 2 fats

1	1-lb. loaf (or round) French bread
½	c. fat-free mayonnaise
2 ½	tsp. Italian seasoning
½	tsp. black pepper
1	tbsp. olive oil
1	onion, chopped
1	red bell pepper, chopped or sliced
1	green bell pepper, chopped or sliced
1	stalk celery, sliced
10	oz. extra-lean ham, thinly sliced
1 ½	c. nonfat cheddar cheese (or nonfat cheddar-mozzarella blend)

2	8-oz. pkgs. fat-free cream cheese, softened
1	8 ½-oz. can crushed pineapple in juice, drained
2	c. chopped pecans
¼	c. finely chopped green bell pepper
2	tbsp. finely chopped onion
1	tsp. seasoned salt

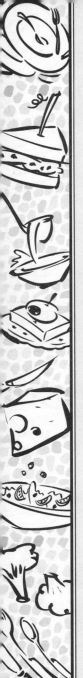

10   6-in. low-fat flour tortillas
2   cucumbers, sliced
2   tomatoes, sliced
1   c. sliced purple onion
1   oz. low-fat feta cheese
1   15-oz. can black beans, drained
1   8-oz. container spicy 3-pepper
     hummus (or flavor of your choice)

10   6-in. low-fat flour tortillas
1   10-oz. pkg. frozen chopped
     spinach, thawed and well drained
1   8-oz. pkg. fat-free cream cheese
1   8-oz. pkg. low-fat sour cream

6   6-in. low-fat flour tortillas
8   oz. fat-free cream cheese
¼   c. chunky salsa

SIMPLE VEGGIE TORTILLAS
Contributed by Tiffany Short, Corpus Christi, Texas

In small bowl, combine cucumbers, tomatoes, onion, cheese and beans; mix well and set aside. Heat tortillas in microwave or on stovetop. For each tortilla, spread 1½ tablespoons hummus on one side; then spoon veggie mixture on top. Roll burrito style and enjoy! Serves 10.
Exchanges: ½ meat, 1½ breads, 1 vegetable, ½ fat

SPINACH WRAPS
Contributed by Karen Israel, Pensacola, Florida

In small bowl, combine spinach, cream cheese and sour cream; mix well. Cover one side of each tortilla with an equal amount of spinach blend; roll tortillas and cut each in half. Cover with plastic wrap and refrigerate several hours. Serves 10.
Exchanges: ½ meat, 1 bread, 1 fat

TORTILLA ROLL-UPS
Contributed by Martha Rogers, Houston, Texas

Mix cream cheese and salsa in small bowl; stir well to combine. Cover one side of each tortilla with an equal amount of cream-cheese blend; roll tortillas and place on serving platter. Cover with plastic wrap and refrigerate at least 1 hour. Slice into 1-inch pieces just prior to serving. Serves 6.
Exchanges: 1 meat, 1 bread

VEGETARIAN QUESADILLAS

Contributed by Johnny Lewis, San Leon, Texas

Coat skillet with cooking spray and sauté vegetables until cooked but still crisp. Place one tortilla on preheated griddle; sprinkle top of tortilla with 2 ounces of cheese. When cheese begins to melt, cover half tortilla with ½ cup sautéed vegetables; fold over and grill until heated through. Slice into three triangle sections to serve. Serve with salsa or picante sauce. Serves 6.

Exchanges: 2 meats, 2 breads, 1 vegetable, 1 fat

6   10-in. low-fat flour tortillas
1 ½ c. thinly sliced onion
1 ½ c. thinly sliced mushrooms
1 ½ c. thinly sliced carrots
1 ½ c. chopped broccoli
12 oz. 2% mozzarella cheese, divided
    Salsa or picante sauce
    Nonstick cooking spray

Tip: You can add 1 ounce chopped chicken breast to each quesadilla. (Add 1 meat exchange.)

BREADS

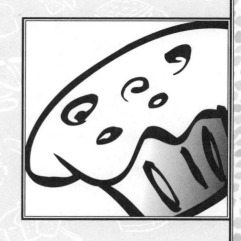

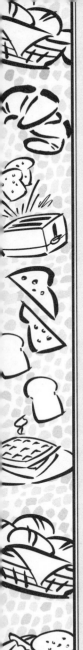

1 c. nonfat milk
2 c. self-rising flour
3 tbsp. fat-free mayonnaise
2 packets artificial sweetener
  (not aspartame)
  Nonstick cooking spray

2 c. all-purpose flour
3 tsp. baking powder
¼ tsp. salt
¼ c. margarine, softened
½ c. milk

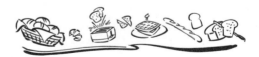

Breads

BISCUITS AND ROLLS

1-2-3 EASY ROLLS
Contributed by Martha Norsworthy, Murray, Kentucky

Preheat oven to 325° F. Combine all ingredients in medium bowl; mix well and spoon into muffin pan coated with cooking spray. Bake 30 minutes. Serves 12.
Exchanges: 1 bread

Tip: Aspartame (e.g., NutraSweet and Equal) loses its sweetness when used for cooking or baking. Acesulfame potassium (e.g., Sunett), saccharin (e.g., Sweet'N Low) and sucralose (e.g., Splenda) all work well in hot foods.

BAKING-POWDER BISCUITS
Contributed by Miriam Rust, Charlotte, North Carolina

Preheat oven to 425° F. Combine flour, baking powder and salt in medium bowl. Cut in margarine; add milk and stir to form a small ball. Roll dough on floured surface to ½ inch thick; cut into 12 equal-sized circles. Bake on ungreased baking sheet 12 to 15 minutes or until tops are golden brown. Serves 12.
Exchanges: 1 bread, 1 fat

EASY ROLLS

Contributed by Carol Moore, Meridian, Mississippi

Combine yeast, flour, salt, water, powdered milk, sugar, oil and egg in large bowl; mix together with large wooden spoon until sticky. Cover with clean cloth and let rise about 45 minutes in a warm place.

After dough has risen, preheat oven to 350° F. Shape dough into 12 rolls and place on baking sheet coated with cooking spray. Spray tops of rolls with light coat of cooking spray; let rise uncovered 30 minutes more. Bake 12 to 15 minutes or until tops are golden brown. Serves 12.

Exchanges: 1 ½ breads, ½ fat

1	pkg. yeast
3 ½	c. all-purpose flour
1	tsp. salt
1 ¼	c. hot water
⅓	c. powdered nonfat milk
¼	c. sugar
2	tbsp. oil
1	egg
	Nonstick cooking spray

LOW-FAT BUTTERMILK BISCUITS

Contributed by Jim Clayton, Lenoir City, Tennessee

Preheat oven to 450° F. In medium bowl, combine flour, oil and buttermilk; mix well. Place dough on waxed paper sprinkled with flour; knead until desired texture and then press down to ½-inch thickness. Cut to create 6 equal-sized circles; place on baking sheet coated with cooking spray. Use cooking spray to coat tops of biscuits; bake 15 minutes or until golden brown. Serves 6.

Exchanges: 1 bread, ½ fat

1	c. self-rising flour
1	tbsp. canola oil
⅓	c. buttermilk
	Butter-flavored nonstick cooking spray

ORANGE ROLLS

Contributed by Judy Marshall, Gilmer, Texas

Preheat oven to 350° F. In shallow dish, combine sugar substitute, orange rind and cinnamon; mix well and set aside. Place orange juice in small bowl; dip each biscuit in juice and then dredge through sugar mixture. Arrange biscuits in 9-inch round baking pan coated with cooking spray. Sprinkle with remaining sugar mixture; drizzle with remaining orange juice. Bake 25 minutes; serve warm. Serves 10.

Exchanges: 1 bread, ½ fat

¼	c. sugar substitute
1 ½	tsp. grated orange rind
½	tsp. cinnamon
3	tbsp. fresh orange juice
10	canned biscuits
	Nonstick cooking spray

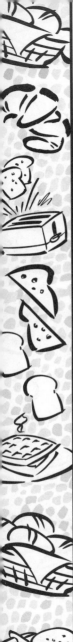

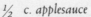

½ c. applesauce
½ c. diced apples
½ c. grated carrots
1 tsp. cinnamon
⅛ tsp. cloves
½ c. Egg Beaters (or other 99% fat-free egg substitute)
6 tbsp. flour
1 tsp. baking powder
⅔ c. powdered milk
10 packets artificial sweetener (not aspartame)
Nonstick cooking spray

2 c. all-purpose flour
1 tbsp. baking powder
¼ tsp. salt
1 tsp. cinnamon
3 packets artificial sweetener (not aspartame)
1 egg
3 tbsp. vegetable oil
½ c. nonfat milk
1 c. unsweetened applesauce
½ c. raisins
Nonstick cooking spray

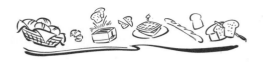

MUFFINS

APPLE-CARROT MUFFINS

Contributed by Patti McCoy, Fort Lupton, Colorado

Preheat oven to 350° F. Combine applesauce, apples, carrots, cinnamon, cloves, egg substitute, flour, baking powder, powdered milk and sweetener in large bowl; mix well and spoon mixture into muffin pan coated with cooking spray. Bake 25 minutes. Serves 6.
Exchanges: ½ fruit, ½ milk, 1 fat

APPLE-RAISIN MUFFINS

Contributed by Mildred Trail, Keswick, Virginia

Preheat oven to 400° F. Coat muffin pan with cooking spray. Combine flour, baking powder, salt, cinnamon and sweetener in large bowl; set aside. In a separate bowl, beat egg; then whip in oil, milk and applesauce. Add to flour mixture and stir until moistened; then stir in raisins. Fill muffin cups each ⅔ full. Bake 25 minutes; remove from pan immediately. Serves 12.
Exchanges: 1 bread, ½ fruit, 1 fat

BANANA MUFFINS

Contributed by Mildred Trail, Keswick, Virginia

Preheat oven to 400° F. Coat muffin pan with cooking spray. In large bowl, beat together egg, oil and milk. Stir in bananas and set aside. In separate bowl, combine flour, baking powder, baking soda and salt; mix well. Stir into banana mixture until flour is moistened. Fill muffin cups each ½ to ⅔ full; bake 23 minutes or until tops are lightly browned. Let cool 15 minutes before removing from pans. Serves 12.

Exchanges: ½ bread, ½ fruit, 1 fat

1 egg
3 tbsp. vegetable oil
¼ c. nonfat milk
1 ⅓ c. mashed bananas
1 c. whole-wheat flour
2 tsp. baking powder
¼ tsp. baking soda
⅛ tsp. salt
Nonstick cooking spray

CHOCOLATE BRAN MUFFINS

Contributed by Janet Kirkhart, Mount Orab, Ohio

Preheat oven to 400° F. Coat muffin pan with cooking spray. Combine cereals in large bowl; set aside. In separate bowl, combine milk with vinegar; add sugar substitute, applesauce, flour, egg whites, baking soda and cocoa. Use large wooden spoon to mix; add to cereal mixture. Fill muffin cups ¾ full; bake 15 minutes. Serves 24.

Exchanges: 1 bread

3 c. Honey Bunches of Oats with Almonds cereal
2 c. Multi-Bran Chex cereal
2 c. Cracklin' Oat Bran cereal
2 ¼ c. nonfat milk
2 tbsp. vinegar
⅓ c. sugar substitute
1 c. unsweetened applesauce
1 c. flour
2 egg whites
3 tsp. baking soda
6 tbsp. cocoa
Nonstick cooking spray

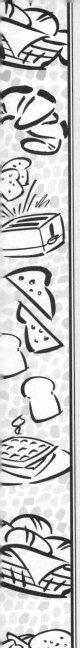

2 c. all-purpose flour
⅔ c. sugar substitute
2 tsp. baking powder
¼ tsp. salt
1 c. fresh cranberries, chopped
⅔ c. nonfat milk
¼ c. reduced-fat margarine, softened
1 tsp. grated orange rind
½ tsp. vanilla extract
1 large egg, lightly beaten
  Nonstick cooking spray

2 eggs
½ c. sugar substitute
¼ c. oil
½ c. orange juice concentrate
½ c. water
2½ c. sifted biscuit mix
¼ c. reduced-sugar orange marmalade
½ c. chopped pecans
  Nonstick cooking spray

FRESH CRANBERRY MUFFINS

Contributed by Martha Norsworthy, Murray, Kentucky

Preheat oven to 400° F. In large bowl, use wire whisk to combine flour, sugar substitute, baking powder and salt. Stir in cranberries; set aside. In separate bowl, combine milk, margarine, orange rind, vanilla extract and egg; stir to blend and add to flour mixture, stirring just until moist. Spoon batter into muffin pan coated with cooking spray; bake 18 minutes or until muffins spring back when touched lightly in center. Remove from pan immediately and place on a wire rack to cool. Serves 12.

Exchanges: 1 bread, ½ fat

Tip: These muffins are freezer friendly! Simply cool completely after baking and store in freezer bags. When ready to use, remove from freezer and thaw at room temperature. Meanwhile, preheat the oven to 300° F. When muffins are thawed, wrap them in aluminum foil and reheat 10 to 15 minutes or until heated through!

ORANGE BLOSSOM MUFFINS

Contributed by Judy Marshall, Gilmer, Texas

Preheat oven to 400° F. Coat miniature-muffin pan with cooking spray. Combine eggs, sugar substitute, oil, orange juice concentrate and water in large bowl; stir well. Add sifted biscuit mix; stir in marmalade and pecans. Let batter sit for a few minutes to rise; fill muffin cups ⅔ full and bake 10 minutes or until golden brown. Serves 24.

Exchanges: ½ bread, 1 fat

SAUSAGE AND CHEESE MUFFINS

Contributed by Patti McCoy, Fort Lupton, Colorado

Preheat oven to 400° F. Preheat skillet coated with cooking spray over medium heat. Cook sausage, bell pepper and onions over low heat until sausage is browned; drain and add jalapeño pepper, if desired. Reduce heat and let simmer. Combine flour, cornmeal, baking soda, salt and red pepper in large bowl; stir well. Form a well in center. Set aside. In a separate bowl, combine buttermilk, margarine and egg; whisk together to blend and then pour into well in dry ingredients, stirring until moistened. Gently fold in sausage mixture and cheese. Spoon batter into muffin pan coated with cooking spray, filling cups ⅔ full. Bake 20 minutes or until tops are golden; remove from pan immediately. Serves 12.
Exchanges: 1 meat, ½ bread, ¾ fat

½ lb. ground sausage
¼ c. chopped green bell pepper
¼ c. chopped green onions
1 tbsp. diced jalapeño pepper (optional)
1 c. all-purpose flour
¼ c. cornmeal
1 tsp. baking soda
¼ tsp. salt
⅛ tsp. ground red pepper
1 c. nonfat buttermilk
2 tsp. margarine, melted
1 large egg, lightly beaten
⅓ c. shredded reduced-fat cheddar cheese
Nonstick cooking spray

TROPICAL MUFFINS

Contributed by Lisa Cramer, Houston, Texas

Preheat oven to 375° F. Sift together flour, sugar substitute, baking powder, baking soda and salt in large bowl. Stir in coconut and form a well in center of mixture; set aside. In separate bowl, combine bananas, margarine, egg, orange rind and orange juice; mix well and pour into dry-ingredients well, stirring until dry ingredients are just moistened. Spoon batter into muffin pan coated with cooking spray, filling cups ⅔ full. Bake 25 to 30 minutes or until lightly browned. Serves 12.
Exchanges: 1 bread, 1 fat

1¾ c. flour
¾ c. sugar substitute
2 tsp. baking powder
¼ tsp. baking soda
½ tsp. salt
¼ c. unsweetened coconut flakes
3 ripe bananas, mashed
⅓ c. reduced-fat margarine, melted
1 egg, beaten
1 tsp. grated orange rind
⅓ c. unsweetened orange juice
Nonstick cooking spray

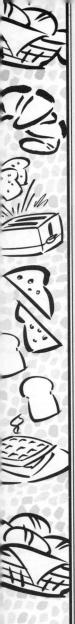

1 c. mashed banana

2 egg whites, or 1 whole jumbo-sized egg

½ c. unsweetened pineapple juice concentrate

¼ c. artificially sweetened vanilla-flavored nonfat yogurt

1 tbsp. water

2 c. low-fat baking mix

2 tsp. baking soda

⅛ tsp. salt

1 c. frozen blueberries, thawed (can also use fresh)

1 packet artificial sweetener (not aspartame)

VERY BERRY BLUEBERRY MUFFINS

Contributed by Lisa Cramer, Houston, Texas

Preheat oven to 350° F. Combine banana, egg whites, pineapple juice concentrate, yogurt and water in large bowl; blend well. Stir in baking mix, baking soda and salt. Gently fold in blueberries; stir 28 to 30 strokes with wooden spoon. Spoon batter into muffin pans lined with muffin liners, filling cups ⅔ full. Bake 20 minutes or until toothpick inserted in center comes out clean. Remove muffins from pan immediately and sprinkle with one packet artificial sweetener, if desired. Serve warm, or cool completely on wire rack and place in airtight container to store. Serves 18.

Exchanges: ½ **bread,** ½ **fruit**

Tip: These muffins will stay fresh in your refrigerator for up to 1 week or in your freezer for up to 2 months!

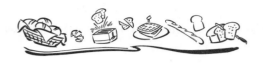

MISCELLANEOUS

BANANA BREAD
Contributed by Carolyn Owen, Charlotte Court House, Virginia

Preheat oven to 350° F. In large bowl, combine banana, sugar substitute, milk, applesauce, oil, vanilla extract and egg whites. Add Bisquick and baking soda; mix well. Pour batter into loaf pan coated with cooking spray. Bake 50 to 60 minutes or until top is lightly browned and toothpick comes out clean. Remove from oven; let sit 10 minutes. Remove from pan and let cool on wire rack (about 2 hours) before slicing. Wrap unused portion tightly with plastic wrap and store in refrigerator. Serves 12.
Exchanges: 1 bread, ½ fruit, ½ fat

Tip: This great bread will stay fresh in your refrigerator for up to 10 days!

½ c. mashed banana
¾ c. sugar substitute
¼ c. nonfat milk
½ c. unsweetened applesauce
1 tsp. oil
¼ tsp. vanilla extract
3 egg whites
2 ½ c. Bisquick baking mix
1 tsp. baking soda
Nonstick cooking spray

BLUE-RIBBON CORNBREAD
Contributed by Kay Smith, Roscoe, Texas

Preheat oven to 425° F. In large bowl, combine cornmeal, flour, salt and baking powder; mix well. Add egg, milk and yogurt; stir to combine and pour into 9x9-inch baking dish coated with cooking spray. Bake 20 minutes. Serves 12.
Exchanges: 1 bread

1 c. cornmeal
1 c. all-purpose flour
½ tsp. salt
1 tbsp. baking powder
1 egg
1 c. nonfat milk
4 oz. artificially sweetened vanilla-flavored nonfat yogurt
Nonstick cooking spray

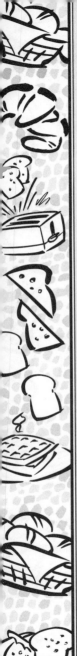

1 ½ c. quick-cooking oats
¼ c. peanut butter
4 pkgs. low-calorie cocoa mix
⅔ c. raisins
2 packets artificial sweetener
¼ c. Grape Nuts cereal
½ c. water
Nonstick cooking spray

2 c. cornmeal
½ tsp. salt
½ tsp. baking soda
2 tsp. baking powder
1 tbsp. honey
1 egg
1 tbsp. vegetable oil
1 c. buttermilk

BREAKFAST BARS
Contributed by Beth Cosby, Lexington, South Carolina

Combine oats, peanut butter, cocoa mix, raisins, sweetener, cereal and water in large bowl; mix well and press into 7x7-inch square baking dish coated with cooking spray. Freeze 30 minutes; cut into bars and wrap individually in plastic wrap. Store in refrigerator or freezer. Serves 6.
Exchanges: 1 bread, ½ milk, ⅔ meat, 1 fruit, 1 fat

BUTTERMILK CORNBREAD
Contributed by Miriam Rust, Charlotte, North Carolina

Preheat oven to 400° F. Lightly coat an 8x8-inch baking dish with oil; set aside. In large bowl, combine cornmeal, salt, baking soda and baking powder; mix well. Stir in honey, egg, oil and milk; blend together and pour into prepared pan. Bake 20 to 25 minutes. Serves 12.
Exchanges: 1 bread

> **Tip:** Out of buttermilk? No problem! Simply combine 1 cup nonfat milk with 1 tablespoon vinegar—voilà!—sour milk. (Great for cooking, but we don't recommend drinkin' it!)

CARROT PATTIES

Contributed by Tammie Bogin, Hendersonville, North Carolina

In small bowl, lightly beat eggs. In medium bowl, combine carrots, celery, onion, bread crumbs, eggs, chervil, salt and pepper. Preheat skillet coated with cooking spray over medium heat. Form carrot patties; cook in skillet 3 to 4 minutes each side or until golden brown. Top each with a dollop of yogurt just prior to serving. Serves 8.

Exchanges: ⅓ bread, ⅓ meat, ⅓ milk

1 ½ c. grated carrots
2 large eggs
¾ c. chopped celery
½ c. onion, excess juice removed by pressing with paper towel
¼ c. bread crumbs
½ c. fresh (or ⅛ c. dried) chervil (can also use parsley)
1 tsp. salt
½ tsp. ground pepper
½ c. plain nonfat yogurt, drained
   Nonstick cooking spray

CHEWY FRUIT-AND-OATMEAL BARS

Contributed by Twila Tillman, Trenton, Missouri

Preheat oven to 350° F. In large bowl, combine sugar substitutes, yogurt, egg whites, applesauce, milk and vanilla extract; mix well and set aside. In medium bowl, combine flour, baking soda, cinnamon and salt; mix well and blend into yogurt mixture. Stir in oats and dried fruit; spread dough into ungreased 9x13-inch baking dish. Bake 28 to 32 minutes or until light golden brown. Cool completely on wire rack; cut into 24 bars and store in a tightly covered container for up to 2 weeks. Serves 24.

Exchanges: 1 bread

¾ c. brown-sugar substitute
½ c. sugar substitute (not aspartame)
1 8-oz. container plain or vanilla-flavored low-fat yogurt
2 egg whites
2 tbsp. applesauce
2 tbsp. nonfat milk
2 tsp. vanilla extract
1 ½ c. all-purpose flour
1 tsp. baking soda
1 tsp. ground cinnamon
½ tsp. salt
3 c. quick-cooking oats (or old-fashioned oats)
1 c. dried raisins, cranberries or mixed fruit

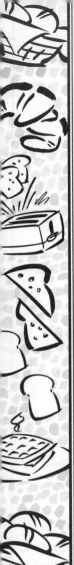

3 c. crumbled **Buttermilk Cornbread**
(see recipe, this section)

1 c. crustless cubed diet bread

2 14½-oz. cans fat-free chicken broth

3 stalks celery, chopped

1 bunch green onions, chopped

¾ c. egg substitute

Poultry seasoning and/or sage to taste

Salt and pepper to taste

Nonstick cooking spray

2 slices diet Italian bread

1 egg

¼ tsp. cinnamon

2 tbsp. nonfat milk

½ tsp. vanilla-butter-and-nut flavoring

1 packet artificial sweetener (not aspartame)

Nonstick cooking spray

CORNBREAD DRESSING

Contributed by Martha Rogers, Houston, Texas

Preheat oven to 350° F. Combine cornbread crumbs, bread cubes, chicken broth, celery, onions, egg substitute, poultry seasoning, salt and pepper in large mixing bowl; mix well (will have soupy consistency). Pour into casserole dish coated with cooking spray. Bake 45 minutes. Serves 10.

Exchanges: ½ meat, 1 bread, 1 fat

FRENCH TOAST

Contributed by Beverly Lowe, Tampa, Florida

Preheat griddle; coat with cooking spray. Combine egg, cinnamon, milk, vanilla-butter-and-nut flavoring and sweetener in shallow dish; beat well with wire whisk. Dredge bread through egg mixture and cook on griddle until golden brown on each side. Serves 1.

Exchanges: 1 bread, 1 meat, ½ fat

Tip: This dish is so yummy that it doesn't even need syrup!

GARLIC-MUSTARD BREAD

Contributed by Martha Rogers, Houston, Texas

Split bread in half lengthwise. In small bowl, mix together margarine, mustard and garlic; spread evenly over bread halves and sprinkle each with sesame seeds. Place under broiler margarine-side up until brown and bubbly. Serves 20.
Exchanges: 1 bread, 1 fat

1 loaf French bread
½ c. reduced-fat margarine, softened
2 tbsp. brown mustard with horseradish
¼ tsp. garlic salt or garlic powder
3 tbsp. sesame seeds

HONEY WHOLE-WHEAT BREAD

Contributed by Sara Wollitz, Callahan, Florida

In bread maker, combine all ingredients in order listed. Set machine on normal, basic or whole-wheat cycle, depending on your machine. Cook approximately 3 hours and enjoy! Serves 16.
Exchanges: 1 bread

....
Tip: This recipe is for your bread-making machine. It's a great way to fill your home with the smell of homemade bread the First Place way!
....

7 ½ oz. water, room temperature
¼ c. honey
1 tbsp. I Can't Believe It's Not Butter spray
1 c. whole-wheat flour
1 c. unbleached flour
1 tsp. salt
1 tbsp. powdered nonfat milk
2 ¼ tsp. active dry yeast

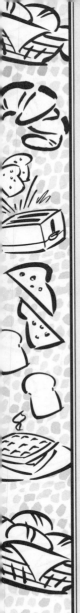

1 ½ c. flour
1 tsp. baking soda
2 tsp. baking powder
2 tbsp. canola oil
3 tbsp. applesauce
1 ¼ c. nonfat milk
3 egg whites
½ c. egg substitute
Nonstick cooking spray

½ c. quick-cooking oats
1 apple, peeled, cored and quartered
1 egg
1 tbsp. artificial sweetener
(not aspartame)
1 tbsp. raisins
1 tsp. vanilla extract
½ tsp. cinnamon
Nonstick cooking spray

LIGHT WAFFLES

Contributed by Sheri Jackson, Okmulgee, Oklahoma

Combine flour, baking soda and baking powder in medium bowl; mix well. Add oil, applesauce, milk, egg whites and egg substitute; stir to combine. Pour onto preheated waffle iron coated with cooking spray; cook until waffle no longer sticks to iron when lid is lifted. Serves 8.

Exchanges: 1 bread, ½ meat, 1 fat

> **Tip:** Substituting an equal amount of applesauce for the oil will remove the fat exchange!

OATMEAL-APPLE PANCAKES

Contributed by Shirlene Hoke, Dallas, North Carolina

Using a blender or food processor, grind oats for a few seconds; pour ground oats into small bowl. Add apple to blender (or food processor); grind until finely chopped and add to bowl. Stir in egg, sweetener, raisins, vanilla extract and cinnamon; mix well. Spoon into 3-inch circles onto preheated griddle coated with cooking spray. Cook until brown on both sides (will have bread-pudding consistency). Serves 1.

Exchanges: 1 meat, 2 breads, 1 ½ fruits, ½ fat

SPINACH BREAD

Contributed by Katina Shelby, New Orleans, Louisiana

Preheat oven to 350° F. Use margarine to sauté onions until tender-crisp. Add chicken bouillon, spinach and cream cheese; stir until smooth. Remove from heat. Spread mix over French bread slices; sprinkle cheese on top. Arrange on shallow baking sheet; bake 10 minutes or until cheese is melted. Serves 15.

Exchanges: 1 bread, ½ meat, ½ vegetable, 1 fat

1   loaf French bread, sliced into
    15 slices
⅔ c. chopped onions
½ c. reduced-fat margarine
2   chicken bouillon cubes
2   10-oz. pkgs. frozen chopped
    spinach
1   8-oz. pkg. light cream cheese
1   c. shredded cheddar cheese
    Granulated garlic to taste

DESSERTS AND SWEETS

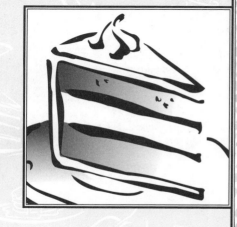

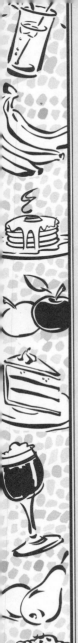

An Important Note

The terms "artificial sweetener" and "sugar substitute" do not refer to the same products in the following recipes! Artificial sweeteners refer to sweeteners measured by the packet (e.g., Equal and Sweet'N Low). Sugar substitutes refer to sweeteners that can be measured as if measuring sugar for cooking or baking (e.g., Splenda).

1   c. nonfat milk
1   c. prepared coffee
1   tsp. vanilla extract
2   tsp. chocolate Ovaltine
1   packet artificial sweetener
    (not aspartame)

1   frozen banana (peel before freezing)
1   c. nonfat milk
1   packet artificial sweetener
1   tbsp. fat-free whipped topping

Desserts and Sweets

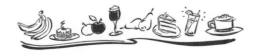

BEVERAGES

ANYTIME CHOCOLATE LATTE

Contributed by Megan Riley, Southport, Florida

Warm milk and coffee in small saucepan using low heat (do not boil). Once warmed (about 3 minutes), pour into mug and stir in vanilla extract, Ovaltine and sweetener. Serves 1.

Exchanges: 1 milk

BANANA MILK SHAKE

Contributed by Jan Jarrett, Hendersonville, North Carolina

Break frozen banana into pieces and place in a blender. Add milk and sweetener; blend until smooth. Serve topped with whipped topping. Serves 1.

Exchanges: 2 fruits, 1 milk

BANANA-BERRY SMOOTHIE

Contributed by Donna Alley, Oxford, Nova Scotia, Canada

Combine juice, yogurt and fruits in blender; add ice and blend until smooth. Serves 1.

Exchanges: 1 milk, 3 fruits

6 oz. unsweetened pineapple juice

6 oz. artificially sweetened plain nonfat yogurt

1 c. frozen berries (any kind)

½ frozen banana, sliced

3 ice cubes

CAPPUCCINO MIX

Contributed by Vicki Mobley, Loganville, Georgia

Combine all ingredients; mix well and store in airtight container. When ready to use, add 3 level tablespoons of mix to 1 ½ cups boiling water. Stir and enjoy! Serves 16.

Exchanges: Free

Tip: Keep a container of this mix handy for entertaining or for when you just want to curl up in your favorite chair and study your Bible!

1 ½ c. powdered fat-free nondairy creamer

½ c. cocoa powder

¾ c. sugar substitute

⅔ c. decaffeinated instant coffee

1 tsp. ground cinnamon

¼ tsp. ground nutmeg

CRANBERRY PUNCH

Contributed by Martha Rogers, Houston, Texas

Completely dissolve gelatin in boiling water; then stir in 1 cup cold water. Add cranberry juice concentrate, pineapple juice, orange juice concentrate, almond extract and remaining water; refrigerate 1 hour or until ready to serve. Add soda prior to serving. Serves 12.

Exchanges: 1 fruit

1 .3-oz. box sugar-free cranberry-flavored gelatin

1 c. boiling water

4 ½ c. cold water, divided

1 12-oz. can light cranberry juice concentrate

32 oz. unsweetened pineapple juice

1 6-oz. can frozen orange juice concentrate

1 tsp. almond extract

2 liters diet ginger ale or lemon-lime soda

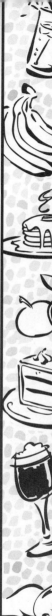

DESSERTS AND SWEETS

Beverages

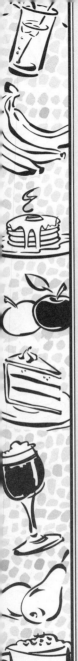

½ c. nonfat milk

1 c. sugar-free vanilla-flavored
   nonfat ice cream

1 tsp. malted milk powder

4 c. cranberry juice cocktail

2 c. orange juice

1 12-oz. can diet lemon-lime soda

½ c. whole cranberries

1 c. frozen strawberries

1 c. nonfat milk

1 packet artificial sweetener

QUICK AND EASY VANILLA MALT

Contributed by Carol Moore, Meridian, Mississippi

This is easy! Simply combine all ingredients in a blender and puree. Serves 1.
Exchanges: 2 breads, ½ milk

Tip: Add 4 strawberries to make a strawberry malt; add 1 to 2 teaspoons fat-free chocolate-flavored ready-to-drink Nesquik for a chocolate malt! (This will not alter the exchanges.)

QUICK CRANBERRY PUNCH

Contributed by Miriam Rust, Charlotte, North Carolina

Combine cranberry and orange juices in large punch bowl. Pour soda down side of bowl; stir and float cranberries on top for garnish. Serves 16.
Exchanges: 1 fruit

STRAWBERRY SMOOTHIE

Contributed by Joy Jarvis, Norcross, Georgia

Use blender to puree all ingredients; pour into glass and enjoy! Serves 1.
Exchanges: 1 milk, 1 fruit

Tip: For a peach smoothie, substitute 1 cup frozen peaches for the strawberries!

TUTTI-FRUTTI SMOOTHIE

Contributed by Pauline Hines, New Orleans, Louisiana

Using a blender on high speed, blend together fruits, juices, smoothie mix, sweetener and ice. Blend until smooth and creamy. Serves 3.

Exchanges: 4 fruits

> **Tip:** You can prepare and freeze the fruit for this smoothie ahead of time. If you choose to do this, omit the 2½ cups crushed ice.

1 apple, chopped
1 pear, chopped
2 cantaloupe wedges, chopped
1 honeydew melon wedge, chopped
1 banana, quartered
1 kiwi, quartered
5 strawberries, halved
1 c. orange juice
1 c. cranberry juice
1 packet powdered yogurt smoothie mix
1 to 2 packets artificial sweetener
2½ c. crushed ice

WASSAIL

Contributed by Martha Rogers, Houston, Texas

Heat cider, brown-sugar substitute and bagged spices in large saucepan. Pour into coffeepot decanter or other heat-resistant serving pot. Serve garnished with orange slices. Serves 16.

Exchanges: 1 fruit

> **Tip:** You can also use your coffee pot to heat this yummy hot beverage.

64 oz. apple cider
½ c. brown-sugar substitute
Cinnamon sticks, whole cloves, allspice in a tea ball or cheesecloth bag
Orange slices for garnish

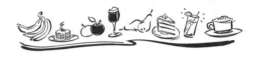

CAKES AND PIES

BANANA-BERRY CREAM PIE
Contributed by Lisa Cramer, Houston, Texas

1 reduced-fat graham-cracker piecrust
1 medium banana, sliced
1 c. sliced strawberries (or other berry)
4 oz. fat-free cream cheese
2 tbsp. strawberry all-fruit spread
3 c. fat-free whipped topping
1 c. nonfat milk
1 .8-oz. box sugar-free vanilla-flavored nonfat instant pudding

Line bottom of piecrust with banana slices; arrange berries over bananas and set aside. Use electric mixer to beat together cream cheese and fruit spread in medium bowl. Gently fold in whipped topping; set aside. In separate bowl, mix milk and pudding until smooth (mixture will be thick). Evenly spread pudding over fruit in piecrust; top with cream cheese mixture and refrigerate at least 3 hours. Serves 8.
Exchanges: ½ **meat, 1 bread,** ½ **fruit,** ½ **fat**

Tip: Although this recipe calls for strawberry all-fruit spread, you can experiment by substituting your favorite all-fruit spread flavors!

BLUEBERRY CHEESECAKE

Contributed by Martha Rogers, Houston, Texas

Preheat oven to 350° F. In medium bowl, combine graham-cracker crumbs with melted margarine, ¼ cup sugar and 4 packets sweetener; mix well and press into bottom of 9x9-inch square baking dish (or 10-inch pie plate) to form crust. Set aside.

Combine cream cheese, eggs, ½ cup sugar and 4 packets sweetener; mix well and pour over pie crust. Bake 15 minutes; remove from oven and cool.

Bring water and blueberries to a boil in saucepan. Remove from heat; strain and reserve juice. Remove blueberries and set aside; return juice to saucepan. Add cornstarch and simmer until juice thickens. Remove from heat; gently stir in blueberries and let cool for 1 hour. Add remaining sweetener and pour cooled mixture over filling in piecrust. Refrigerate 2 hours before serving. Serves 14.

Exchanges: 1 bread, ½ fat, ½ fruit, ¼ meat

- 16 low-fat graham crackers, crushed
- ¼ c. margarine, melted
- ¾ c. sugar, divided
- 12 packets artificial sweetener (not aspartame)
- 8 oz. fat-free cream cheese
- 2 eggs
- 1 c. water
- 1 ½ c. blueberries (fresh or frozen)
- 2 tbsp. cornstarch

CHOCOLATE AND PEANUT BUTTER CHEESECAKE PIE

Contributed by Debbie Vanlandingham, Ovilla, Texas

Line bottom of 8x8-inch baking dish with 8 crackers; set aside. Soften gelatin using cold milk in small microwave-safe bowl for about 5 minutes; stir and add pudding mix. Microwave 2 minutes; stir and continue to cook and stir until pudding thickens. Remove from microwave; use wire whisk to stir in peanut butter and cream cheese until well blended. Allow to cool thoroughly, stirring occasionally. Gently fold in whipped topping; pour into pan lined with graham crackers. Refrigerate at least 4 hours. Serves 8.

Exchanges: 1 bread, ½ meat, ½ milk, ½ fat

- 8 low-fat graham crackers
- 1 envelope plain gelatin
- 2 c. nonfat milk
- 1 1.4-oz. box sugar-free chocolate-flavored nonfat instant pudding
- 3 tbsp. peanut butter
- 8 oz. fat-free cream cheese
- 1 c. fat-free whipped topping

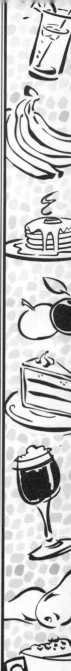

8   graham crackers, divided into
     16 pieces
1   1.4-oz. box sugar-free white-
     chocolate-flavored nonfat instant
     pudding
1   1.4-oz. box sugar-free chocolate-
     flavored nonfat instant pudding
3 ½ c. nonfat milk, divided
2   bananas, sliced
3   c. fat-free whipped topping

1   .8-oz. box sugar-free vanilla-
     flavored nonfat instant pudding
⅔   c. powdered nonfat milk
1   c. water
½   tsp. mint extract
     Green food coloring
1   c. reduced-fat whipped topping
2   tbsp. miniature chocolate chips
1   6-oz. chocolate-wafer piecrust

CHOCOLATE BANANA CREAM PIE

Contributed by Martha Rogers, Houston, Texas

Line a pie plate (or oblong baking dish) with graham-cracker pieces; set aside. Prepare puddings in separate bowls, mixing each with 1 ¾ cup milk and whipping until set. Pour white-chocolate pudding over top of graham crackers; layer with banana slices and top with chocolate pudding. Refrigerate 2 hours or until set. Top with whipped topping prior to serving. Serves 8.
Exchanges: ½ bread, ½ milk, ½ fruit

CHOCOLATE MINT PIE

Contributed by Joe Ann Winkler, Overland Park, Kansas

Combine pudding mix, powdered milk and water; mix well using a wire whisk. Add mint extract, 2 drops food coloring and whipped topping; stir in chocolate chips. Pour mixture into piecrust; refrigerate until ready to serve. Serves 8.
Exchanges: 1 bread, 2 fats

CREAMY PUMPKIN SOUFFLÉ

Contributed by Lisa Cramer, Houston, Texas

Combine pudding mix and milk in medium bowl; stir well. Add pumpkin, nutmeg, ginger and cinnamon; stir. Gently fold in whipped topping; pour into pudding cups. Refrigerate 1 hour or until set. Serves 8.
Exchanges: ½ bread

Tip: Serve as pumpkin pie by pouring the mixture into a reduced-fat grahamcracker piecrust. (Add 1 bread and 1 fat to exchanges.)

---

1   1½-oz. box sugar-free vanilla-flavored nonfat instant pudding
1   c. nonfat milk
1   16-oz. can pumpkin
½   tsp. nutmeg
½   tsp. ginger
½   tsp. cinnamon
1   c. fat-free whipped topping

FRUIT DELIGHT CHEESECAKE

Contributed by Carol Moore, Meridian, Mississippi

Line bottom of 11x7-inch baking dish with graham crackers; add layer of banana slices and set aside. In large bowl, beat together cream cheese and ½ cup milk with a wire whisk until smooth. Stir in remaining 1½ cups milk and pudding mix; beat with wire whisk 1 minute. Stir in whipped topping until smooth and well blended. Spoon mixture into dish over top of banana slices; garnish with colorful fruit. Refrigerate 4 hours or until set. Serves 8.
Exchanges: 1 bread, ½ meat, ½ fruit, ¼ milk

Tip: This makes a beautiful dessert for a luau or other summer celebrations. You can even use a red-white-and-blue theme for Independence Day!

---

6   low-fat graham crackers
2   bananas, sliced (or 2 c. canned fruit of choice, well-drained)
8   oz. fat-free cream cheese, softened
2   c. nonfat milk, divided
2   1.4-oz. boxes sugar-free white-chocolate-flavored nonfat instant pudding
3   c. fat-free whipped topping, thawed
    Fruit for garnish (not bananas)

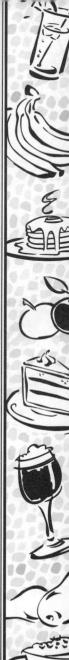

DESSERTS AND SWEETS

Cakes and Pies

1 envelope plain gelatin
3 tbsp. lime juice
½ c. boiling water
1 packet artificial sweetener
1 c. evaporated nonfat milk
1 tsp. vanilla extract
1 tbsp. lime juice
Green food coloring
1 9-in. low-fat graham-cracker piecrust
Lime zest for garnish
1 lime, thinly sliced, for garnish

KEY LIME PIE

Contributed by Pam Danford, Ashford, Alabama

Sprinkle gelatin over 3 tablespoons lime juice in small bowl; let stand 1 minute and then add boiling water and sweetener. Stir until gelatin is dissolved; refrigerate 45 minutes or until slightly thickened.

Approximately 10 to 15 minutes after placing gelatin in refrigerator, combine milk and vanilla extract in freezer-safe container and place in freezer 30 minutes. Remove from freezer and whip at high speed until stiff. Stir in 1 tablespoon lime juice and 2 drops food coloring. Remove gelatin from refrigerator and slowly blend into whipped milk. Spoon mixture into piecrust; refrigerate 4 hours or until firm. Garnish with lime zest and several lime slices. Serves 8.

Exchanges: ½ milk, 1 ½ fats, 1 ½ breads

LEMON-CHERRY CHEESECAKE

Contributed by Debbie Vanlandingham, Ovilla, Texas

Line bottom of 8x8-inch baking dish with graham crackers; set aside. Combine gelatin and cold water; stir and set aside. Use microwave-safe cup to heat remaining water 2 minutes in microwave; stir into cold gelatin mixture and set aside to cool. In small bowl, combine yogurt and cream cheese; blend with back of spoon until well mixed; set aside. Combine pudding mix, powdered milk and gelatin mixture in large bowl; whip using a wire whisk until thickened. Fold in yogurt mixture and whipped topping until well blended; pour over graham crackers. Refrigerate at least 4 hours.

Combine cherries, tapioca, sugar substitute, almond extract and few drops food coloring in microwave-safe dish; microwave 10 minutes, stirring twice during cooking. Remove from microwave and cool completely. Spoon mixture evenly over top of cold pie and chill until ready to serve. Serves 8.

Exchanges: 1 bread, ½ meat, ½ milk

8	low-fat graham crackers
1	envelope plain gelatin
¼	c. cold water
¾	c. room temperature water
6	oz. artificially sweetened lemon-flavored low-fat yogurt
4	oz. fat-free cream cheese
1	1.4-oz. box sugar-free white-chocolate-flavored nonfat instant pudding
⅔	c. powdered nonfat milk
1	c. light whipped topping
1	21-oz. can cherry pie filling
1	tbsp. tapioca
¾	c. sugar substitute
1	tsp. almond extract
	Red food coloring

MINICHEESECAKES

Contributed by Jan Jarrett, Hendersonville, North Carolina

Preheat oven to 350° F. Coat 3 miniature-muffin pans (36 muffins total) with nonstick cooking spray; set aside. In medium bowl, blend together cream cheeses and egg substitute; mix well. Stir in sweetener, lemon juice and vanilla extract. Fill muffin cups half full; bake 15 minutes or until slightly brown. Allow to cool 10 minutes; remove from pan and refrigerate for 2 hours. Top each cheesecake with 1 teaspoon all-fruit spread prior to serving. Serves 12.

Exchanges: ½ meat, ½ fruit, ½ fat

8	oz. fat-free cream cheese
8	oz. light cream cheese
½	c. egg substitute
4 to 5	packets artificial sweetener (not aspartame)
2	tbsp. lemon juice
½	tsp. vanilla extract
¾	c. all-fruit spread
	Nonstick cooking spray

Tip: Use a flat icing knife to remove cooled cheesecakes from muffin cups.

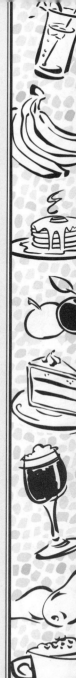

2 c. fresh or frozen peaches (can substitute blackberries or raspberries)
1 tsp. ground cinnamon
1 tsp. lemon juice
1 c. all-purpose flour
1 ½ c. sugar substitute, divided
1 tsp. baking powder
½ c. nonfat milk
3 tbsp. fat-free liquid margarine
1 tbsp. cornstarch
1 c. boiling water
Nonstick cooking spray

1 9-in. frozen piecrust, thawed
4 tbsp. unsweetened applesauce
1 tsp. brown-sugar substitute
¼ tsp. cinnamon
2 medium apples
(tart apples are best), sliced thin
1 tsp. lemon juice
2 tbsp. apricot all-fruit spread, warmed

PEACH PUDDING CAKE

Contributed by Carolyn Owen, Charlotte Court House, Virginia

Preheat oven to 350° F. In small bowl, toss peaches with cinnamon and lemon juice; arrange in 8x8-inch baking dish coated with cooking spray and set aside. In medium bowl, combine flour, ¾ cup sugar substitute and baking powder; mix well. Stir in milk and margarine; spoon evenly over fruit in baking dish. In small bowl, combine remaining sugar substitute with cornstarch; sprinkle over milk-margarine mixture. Slowly pour boiling water over top; bake 45 to 50 minutes or until toothpick comes out clean. Serves 4.

Exchanges: 1 bread, ½ fruit

Tip: This is delicious served warm with ¼ cup sugar-free vanilla-flavored nonfat ice cream! (Add 1 bread exchange.)

PIE-PAN APPLE TART

Contributed by Sheila Robbins, Houston, Texas

Preheat oven to 350° F. Place piecrust into an 8-inch pie plate and push dough halfway down sides to form a thick crust around edge; pinch top and push finger against side to form crimped and pleated edge. Prick bottom with a fork; bake 10 minutes and cool slightly. Spread applesauce over bottom of piecrust; sprinkle brown-sugar substitute and cinnamon over top. Arrange apple slices over applesauce; sprinkle apples with lemon juice. Coat top with warmed all-fruit spread; bake 30 to 35 minutes. Serves 6.

Exchanges: ½ bread, ½ fruit, 1 fat

PINEAPPLE-COCONUT PIE

Contributed by Martha Rogers, Houston, Texas

In small bowl, combine pudding mix and milk; blend until thick. Stir in coconut and pineapple; pour mixture into pie shell and refrigerate at least 2 hours. Garnish each piece with 3 tablespoons whipped topping. Serves 8.
Exchanges: 1 bread, ½ fruit, 1½ fats

- 1 .8-oz. box sugar-free vanilla-flavored nonfat instant pudding
- 1 c. nonfat milk
- ½ c. flaked coconut
- 1 8-oz. can pineapple chunks in juice, drained
- 1 8-in. pie shell, cooked and cooled
- 1½ c. fat-free whipped topping

STRAWBERRY TRIFLE

Contributed by Becky Sirt, The Woodlands, Texas

Line bottom of 9x13-inch baking dish with cake pieces; set aside. Dissolve gelatin in water; add strawberries (with juice) to gelatin; spoon mixture evenly over cake pieces. Slice bananas on top and refrigerate. Prepare pudding as directed on package using nonfat milk. Pour pudding over bananas; top with whipped topping and refrigerate 1 to 2 hours. Garnish with sliced fresh strawberries, if available. Serves 15.
Exchanges: 1 bread, ½ fruit, ½ fat

....

Tip: A pancake turner works great for serving this dessert!

....

- ½ large prepared angel-food cake, torn into bite-sized pieces
- 1 .3-oz. box sugar-free strawberry-flavored gelatin
- 1 c. water, boiling
- 1 9-oz. pkg. frozen strawberries, thawed
- 2 large bananas
- 2 .8-oz. boxes sugar-free vanilla-flavored nonfat instant pudding
- 4½ c. light whipped topping

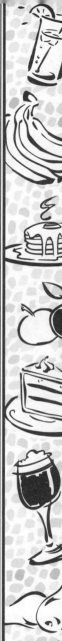

1   6-oz. can frozen apple juice
    concentrate, undiluted
1   tbsp. cornstarch
3   tbsp. light butter
1   tsp. cinnamon
4   c. peeled and sliced apples
2   piecrust sheets

1   c. water
1   c. raisins
1   c. diced unsweetened dried fruit
2   c. flour
1   c. sugar substitute
1 ½   tsp. ground cinnamon
1   tsp. baking soda
½   tsp. salt
½   tsp. ground nutmeg
½   c. egg substitute
1   c. unsweetened applesauce
½   c. vegetable oil
1   tsp. vanilla extract
½   c. chopped nuts
       Nonstick cooking spray

SUGAR-FREE APPLE PIE

Contributed by Julia Faulk, Louisville, Mississippi

Preheat oven to 400° F. Heat apple juice concentrate in medium saucepan; add cornstarch and bring to boil for about 30 seconds. Remove from heat; stir in butter and cinnamon. Add apples and stir until well coated; pour into piecrust placed in pan and cover with second piecrust sheet. Bake 45 to 50 minutes. Serves 8.
Exchanges: 2 breads, ½ fruit, 1 ½ fats

SUGAR-FREE APPLESAUCE CAKE

Contributed by Beth Cosby, Lexington, South Carolina

Preheat oven to 325° F. In a saucepan, bring water to a boil. Add raisins and dried fruit; remove from heat and let stand 10 minutes. Drain well and set aside. Combine flour, sugar substitute, cinnamon, baking soda, salt and nutmeg in large bowl; mix well and set aside. In separate bowl, combine egg substitute, applesauce, oil and vanilla extract until blended. Stir into dry ingredients until well blended. Fold in nuts and fruit mixture. Pour into loaf pan coated with cooking spray. Bake 35 to 40 minutes or until a toothpick inserted near the center of the cake comes out clean. Cool in pan 10 minutes before removing to a wire rack. Serves 16.
Exchanges: ½ bread, 1 ½ fruits, 2 fats

SUGAR-FREE STRAWBERRY PIE

Contributed by Alyce Amussen, Silver Spring, Maryland

Combine gelatin mix, pudding mix and cold water in small saucepan; cook over medium heat until boiling, stirring constantly. Remove from heat; pour into medium bowl and refrigerate 30 to 60 minutes or until slightly thickened. Once thickened, stir in strawberries and pour into piecrust; refrigerate 4 hours or until set. Serves 8.
Exchanges: 1 bread, ½ fruit, 1 fat

1 .3-oz. box sugar-free strawberry-flavored gelatin

1 .8-oz. box sugar-free vanilla-flavored nonfat pudding

3 c. cold water

4 c. sliced strawberries

1 9-in. piecrust, baked and cooled

THREE-LAYER APPLE-RAISIN PIE

Contributed by Kay Smith, Roscoe, Texas

In a medium saucepan, combine 3 cups water and apples; let soak 3 to 5 minutes; then simmer over low heat 30 minutes. Stir in raisins and cinnamon; cook 15 minutes more. Dissolve cornstarch in ¼ cup water and add to apple mixture; cook 5 minutes more and set aside to cool.

　　After apples have cooled, add sweetener and pour mixture into piecrust; set aside. In small bowl, prepared pudding mix according to package directions; blend well and pour over apple filling. Refrigerate at least 1 hour; top with whipped topping prior to serving. Serves 8.
Exchanges: 1¼ breads, 1 fruit, ½ milk, 1½ fats

3¼ c. water, divided

1 5-oz. bag dried apple pieces

½ c. raisins

1 tsp. cinnamon

1 tsp. cornstarch

4 packets artificial sweetener

1 piecrust, cooked and cooled

1 1½-oz. box sugar-free vanilla-flavored nonfat instant pudding

2 c. fat-free whipped topping

WHITE-CHOCOLATE CHEESECAKE

Contributed by Melba Rodgers, Duck Hill, Mississippi

Use wire whisk to beat together cream cheese and ½ cup milk in medium bowl. Add remaining milk and pudding mixes; whisk for 1 minute. Stir in whipped topping and blend until smooth. Spoon equal amounts of mixture into each pie crust. Refrigerate 4 hours or until set. Serves 16.
Exchanges: ½ meat, 1 bread, 1 fat

1 8-oz. container fat-free cream cheese

2 c. nonfat milk, divided

2 1.4-oz. boxes sugar-free white-chocolate-flavored nonfat instant pudding

3 c. fat-free whipped topping

2 6-oz. graham-cracker-crumb piecrusts

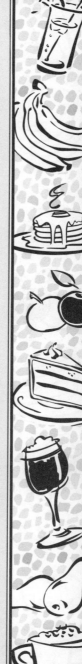

FROZEN TREATS

BLUE-RIBBON FROZEN SNICKER DESSERT
Contributed by Lisa Cramer, Houston, Texas

Press graham-cracker crumbs into an 8x8-inch baking dish; set aside. In large bowl, combine frozen yogurt, whipped topping, peanut butter and pudding mix; stir well and pour into pan, being careful not to disturb the crumbs. Freeze 2 hours or until firm. Let thaw 10 minutes before serving. Serves 8.
Exchanges: ½ meat, 1 bread, ½ fat

½ c. graham-cracker crumbs

12 oz. artificially sweetened vanilla-flavored nonfat frozen yogurt (or fat-free ice cream)

1 c. fat-free whipped topping

3 tbsp. chunky peanut butter

1 1.4-oz. box sugar-free chocolate-flavored nonfat instant pudding

CHOCOLATE ICE CREAM
Contributed by Connie Armstrong, Hattiesburg, Mississippi

Use electric mixer to blend together pudding mix, sweetener, cocoa powder, evaporated milk and vanilla extract in medium bowl. Fold in whipped topping; stir until smooth and pour into ice-cream-maker container. Add milk; stir until well blended. Freeze according to ice-cream-maker instructions. Serves 32.
Exchanges: ½ milk

1 pkg. sugar-free chocolate-flavored nonfat instant pudding

6 packets artificial sweetener

2 tbsp. cocoa powder

4½ c. evaporated nonfat milk

1 tsp. vanilla extract

3 c. fat-free whipped topping, thawed

5 c. nonfat milk

FROZEN PINEAPPLE-BANANA CUPS

Contributed by Kathy Israel, Pensacola, Florida

1	16-oz. container light sour cream
2	tbsp. lemon juice
⅛	tsp. salt
¾	c. sugar substitute
1	20-oz. can crushed pineapple in juice, drained
3	medium bananas, diced
12	maraschino cherries

Line muffin pan with foil baking cups; set aside. In medium bowl, combine sour cream, lemon juice, salt and sugar substitute. Gently stir in pineapple and banana pieces. Fill baking cups with mixture; add cherry to top of each. Freeze 4 hours or until firm. Once frozen, remove from muffin pan and store in large freezer bag. Thaw 15 to 20 minutes before serving. Serves 12.
Exchanges: 1 fruit, 1 fat

Tip: This is a versatile dish! As a salad with dinner, serve on lettuce leaves; as a dessert, serve in dessert dishes.

HOMEMADE CHOCOLATE ICE CREAM

Contributed by Carol Moore, Meridian, Mississippi

4	eggs, beaten
2	12-oz. cans evaporated nonfat milk
2	tsp. vanilla extract
1	2.1-oz. box sugar-free chocolate-flavored nonfat instant pudding
1	1.4-oz. box sugar-free chocolate-flavored nonfat instant pudding
2	c. nonfat milk
4	packets artificial sweetener

In large bowl, combine eggs, evaporated milk and vanilla extract; slowly whisk in both chocolate-pudding mixes. Pour immediately into ice-cream-maker container; add nonfat milk to full mark and mix. Freeze according to ice-cream-maker instructions. Add sweetener to taste. Serves 16.
Exchanges: ½ meat, ½ milk

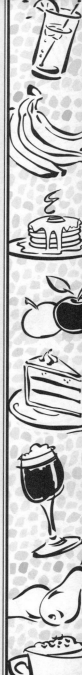

6 low-fat graham crackers
1 1½-oz. box sugar-free vanilla-
   flavored nonfat instant pudding
½ .8-g. container Crystal Light
   sugar-free lemonade drink mix
2 c. nonfat milk
3 c. fat-free whipped topping, divided

1 envelope plain gelatin
¼ c. frozen orange juice concentrate,
   thawed
2 tbsp. sugar
½ tsp. vanilla extract
½ c. nonfat powdered milk
½ c. cold water
1 tbsp. lemon juice
24 low-fat graham crackers

LEMON ICEBOX DESSERT
Contributed by Lisa Cramer, Houston, Texas

Line bottom of 11x7-inch baking dish with graham crackers; set aside. In a large bowl, use electric mixer on low speed to blend together pudding mix, lemonade mix and milk. Use spatula or wooden spoon to fold in 2¼ cups of whipped topping. Pour mixture over graham crackers; top with remaining whipped topping. Refrigerate until ready to serve. Serves 8.
Exchanges: 1 bread, ½ milk

LIGHT AND LUSCIOUS ORANGE BARS
Contributed by Patti McCoy, Fort Lupton, Colorado

Place a small mixing bowl and beaters from electric mixer into refrigerator to chill Soften gelatin in orange juice concentrate using top section of double boiler, stirring completely over boiling water in bottom section. Remove from heat and stir in sugar and vanilla extract. In chilled bowl, combine powdered milk and cold water; use chilled beaters to beat until soft peaks form. Add lemon juice and beat until stiff; fold in juice mixture. Spread evenly on 12 graham crackers; top with remaining graham crackers. Wrap individually in plastic wrap; freeze 2 hours or until firm. Serves 12.
Exchanges: ½ bread

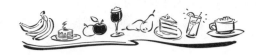

GELATIN TREATS

APPLE SALAD MOLD

Contributed by Lisa Cramer, Houston, Texas

Combine apple juice with cold water; set aside. Dissolve gelatin in boiling water; stir in juice mixture. Refrigerate 1½ hours or until slightly thickened. Stir in apples and celery; mix well and return to refrigerator. Chill 4 hours or until set. Serves 5.
Exchanges: ½ fruit

....
Tip: Although this recipe calls for cherry-flavored gelatin, you can also experiment by substituting other gelatin flavors to suit your taste!
....

½ c. apple juice
½ c. cold water
1 .3 oz. box sugar-free cherry-flavored gelatin
   (or alternate flavor)
1 c. boiling water
1 medium apple, peeled and chopped
½ c. celery

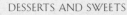

2 c. water

4 oz. fat-free cream cheese

2 .3-oz. boxes sugar-free lime-flavored gelatin

1 c. ice cubes

1 ½ c. fat-free whipped topping

1 8-oz. can crushed pineapple in juice

4 pecan halves, chopped

3 c. fat-free whipped topping

1 16-oz. pkg. frozen strawberries

1 16-oz. container fat-free cottage cheese, drained

1 .3-oz. box sugar-free gelatin, flavor of your choice

1 8-oz. can pineapple tidbits, drained

COOL LIME GELATIN

Contributed by Judy Marshall, Gilmer, Texas

Combine water and cream cheese in microwave-safe bowl; microwave on high 4 minutes. Stir well; whisk in gelatin until dissolved and cream cheese is no longer visible. Add ice cubes and whipped topping; whisk until mixed. Stir in pineapple (with juice); pour into 7x11-inch glass baking dish. Garnish with chopped pecans; chill 4 hours or until set. Serves 8.

Exchanges: ½ fruit

Tip: This recipe is versatile! Use your favorite gelatin flavors and fruits to create some wonderful treats. Here are just a few suggestions:
- Peach-flavored gelatin and chopped peaches, canned in own juice
- Strawberry-flavored gelatin and sliced strawberries (add ½ cup water)
- Orange- or lemon-flavored gelatin and mandarin oranges

FRUIT FLUFF

Contributed by Melba S. Hudson, Orange, Texas

Combine all ingredients in large serving dish; mix well. Cover and refrigerate several hours. Serves 8.

Exchanges: 1 meat, ½ fruit

PUDDINGS

CHOCOLATE-MOCHA MOUSSE
Contributed by Judy Marshall, Gilmer, Texas

Use wire whisk to blend together pudding mix and milk in medium bowl; set aside. In separate bowl, combine whipped topping and coffee mix; set aside. Spoon half the pudding mixture into 4 parfait glasses; cover with a dollop of mocha topping; then top with remaining pudding mixture. Refrigerate until ready to serve. Serves 4.

Exchanges: ½ **milk**

1   1.4-oz. box sugar-free chocolate-flavored nonfat instant pudding
2   c. nonfat milk
1   c. fat-free whipped topping
1   tbsp. sugar-free Swiss-mocha-flavored instant coffee mix

FIRST PLACE BANANA PUDDING
Contributed by Lisa Cramer, Houston, Texas

Sprinkle graham-cracker crumbs on bottom of 13x9-inch baking dish; layer banana slices over crumbs and set aside. Use small bowl to combine pudding and milk; pour pudding over banana slices. Spread whipped topping on top; refrigerate until ready to serve. Serves 6.

Exchanges: ½ **bread, 1 fruit,** ½ **milk**

¾   c. low-fat graham-cracker crumbs
3   bananas, sliced
1   .9-oz. box sugar-free banana-flavored nonfat instant pudding
2   c. nonfat milk
1   c. fat-free whipped topping

2 envelopes plain gelatin
2 tbsp. cold water
2 ¼ c. evaporated nonfat milk, divided
1 ½ c. canned pumpkin
6 tbsp. brown-sugar substitute
1 tsp. pumpkin-pie spice
1 tsp. vanilla extract
Nonstick cooking spray

1 c. reduced-calorie cranberry-
grape juice
2 .3-oz. boxes sugar-free raspberry-
flavored gelatin
1 16-oz. can jellied cranberry sauce
4 c. fat-free whipped topping, thawed

LIGHT AND EASY NO-CRUST PUMPKIN PIE

Contributed by Patti McCoy, Fort Lupton, Colorado

In a medium bowl, sprinkle gelatin over cold water to soften; set aside. In small saucepan, heat 1 ½ cups evaporated milk to just boiling (do not bring to full boil); remove from heat and slowly stir into gelatin until dissolved. Stir in remaining evaporated milk, pumpkin, brown-sugar substitute, pumpkin-pie spice and vanilla extract. Pour mixture into 10-inch pie plate coated with cooking spray; refrigerate 4 hours or until firm. Serves 8.

Exchanges: ½ bread, ½ milk

LIGHT CRANBERRY MOUSSE

Contributed by Laura Hartness, Kernersville, North Carolina

Heat cranberry-grape juice to boiling in small saucepan; remove from heat. Add gelatin, stirring constantly until dissolved; set aside. In medium bowl, beat cranberry sauce using electric mixer on high 1 minute; add gelatin mixture and refrigerate 1 ½ hours or until thickened but not set. Using a rubber spatula, gently fold in whipped topping; spoon into parfait cups and refrigerate 4 hours or until firm. Keep refrigerated in covered container until ready to serve. Serves 10.

Exchanges: 1 bread

RICH AND CREAMY BANANA PUDDING

Contributed by Lynda Martinaz, Madison, Mississippi

In a large bowl, combine milk and pudding mix; stir until thick. Add sour cream and whipped topping. Mix well. In a large serving dish, layer vanilla wafers, sliced bananas and pudding mix. Continue to layer until all pudding is used. Top with a layer of wafers. Refrigerate several hours before serving. Serves 16.
Exchanges: ½ bread, ½ fruit, ½ milk, ½ fat

3   c. nonfat milk

2   .8-oz. boxes sugar-free vanilla-
    or banana-flavored nonfat instant
    pudding

1   8-oz. container fat-free sour cream

3   c. fat-free whipped topping

1   11-oz. box reduced-fat vanilla
    wafers

5 or 6   bananas, sliced

TROPICAL PUDDING

Contributed by Martha Rogers, Houston, Texas

Line bottom of 8x8-inch baking dish with graham crackers; set aside. Cook pudding according to package directions but using only 2 cups milk; remove from heat and allow to cool. Add yogurt, pineapple and banana; fold in half the whipped topping. Pour mixture over graham crackers in dish; top with remaining whipped topping and garnish with mandarin orange slices. Serves 6.
Exchanges: 1 bread, ½ fruit

3   low-fat graham crackers, broken
    into 12 rectangles

1   1½-oz. box sugar-free vanilla-
    flavored nonfat pudding

2   c. nonfat milk

1   8-oz. container Light Yoplait
    Orange Crème Yogurt

1   8-oz. can pineapple chunks in juice

1   banana, chopped

3   c. fat-free whipped topping

1   10½-oz. can mandarin oranges

6 medium apples, peeled, cored and thinly sliced

1 6-oz. can frozen apple juice concentrate, unsweetened and undiluted

2 tbsp. cornstarch

3 tbsp. reduced-fat margarine, divided

1 tsp. cinnamon

1 tsp. vanilla extract

½ c. flour

⅛ tsp. salt

⅛ tsp. nutmeg

1 apple, peeled and sliced

1 tsp. orange juice

2 tsp. sugar substitute

2 tbsp. crushed cornflakes

1 tsp. reduced-fat margarine

MISCELLANEOUS

APPLE COBBLER

Contributed by Lisa Cramer, Houston, Texas

Preheat oven to 350° F. In a medium saucepan, combine apple juice and cornstarch; cook over medium heat until thick and bubbly. Stir in 1 tablespoon margarine, cinnamon and vanilla extract; add apples and toss to coat. Pour into 9-inch pie plate; set aside. In a separate bowl, mix together flour, salt, nutmeg and 2 tablespoons margarine until crumbly; sprinkle over apple mixture. Bake 30 minutes. Excellent served warm. Serves 8.

Exchanges: 1 ½ fruits, ½ bread, ½ fat

APPLE CRISP

Contributed by Patti McCoy, Fort Lupton, Colorado

Preheat oven to 350° F. Place apple slices in small baking dish. Sprinkle with orange juice, sugar substitute and crushed cornflakes; top with margarine. Bake 20 to 25 minutes. Serves 1.

Exchanges: 1 ½ fruits, 1 fat

Tip: In a hurry? Microwave your apple crisp instead of baking it. Simply microwave on high 2 to 3 minutes in a microwave-safe dish; let sit 2 minutes and enjoy!

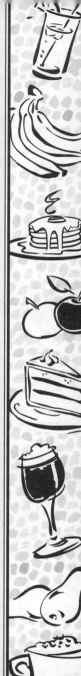

APPLE DESSERT

Contributed by Susan Gehrum, Turbotville, Pennsylvania

In small bowl, prepare pudding using 1½ cups milk instead of 2 cups called for in box directions. Refrigerate 30 minutes or until set; then remove and fold in whipped topping, apples and cranberries. Just prior to serving, sprinkle granola on top (granola will get soggy if mixed in too early before serving). Serves 16.
Exchanges: ½ bread, ½ fruit

1	.8-oz. box sugar-free vanilla-flavored nonfat instant pudding
1½	c. nonfat milk
1½	c. fat-free whipped topping
3	c. chopped apples
⅔	c. dried cranberries
2	pkgs. (4 bars) honey-and-oat granola bars, crumbled

BAKED APPLES

Contributed by Geneva Reed, Camden, Tennessee

Preheat oven to 350° F. Arrange apples in baking dish; pour water over apples and sprinkle with dry gelatin. Bake 30 minutes or until tender. Serves 6.
Exchanges: 1 fruit

6	medium apples, peeled and cored
1	c. water
1	.3 oz. box sugar-free strawberry-flavored gelatin

BANANA-SPLIT DESSERT

Contributed by Lisa Cramer, Houston, Texas

Line bottom of 13x9-inch baking dish with 8 graham crackers; set aside. In large bowl, combine banana pudding and 3 cups milk; mix well and let sit 2 minutes. Stir in pineapple chunks; then gently fold in whipped topping. Pour half the mixture into baking dish; reserve remainder. Arrange banana slices over pudding mixture; add layer of 8 graham crackers. Pour in remaining pudding mixture; add layer of sliced strawberries and top with remaining graham crackers. Set aside. In separate bowl, combine chocolate pudding with 1½ cups milk; mix well and let sit 2 minutes. Spread as topping over graham crackers. Refrigerate at least 6 hours to soften graham crackers; garnish with chopped pecans prior to serving. Serves 18.
Exchanges: 1 bread, ¼ milk, ½ fruit

24	low-fat graham crackers
2	.9-oz. boxes sugar-free banana-flavored nonfat instant pudding
4½	c. nonfat milk, divided
1	16-oz. can crushed pineapple, drained
3¾	c. fat-free whipped topping, thawed
2	bananas, sliced
2	c. sliced strawberries
1	1.4-oz. box sugar-free chocolate-flavored nonfat instant pudding
2	tbsp. chopped pecans

Blue-Ribbon Brownies
(see recipe, this section)

1   1½-oz. box sugar-free vanilla-
    flavored nonfat instant pudding
1   2.1 oz. box sugar-free chocolate-
    flavored nonfat instant pudding
3   c. light whipped topping
¼   c. chopped pecans

1½   c. Pioneer brand nonfat baking mix
8   oz. vanilla- or caramel-flavored
     low-fat yogurt
4   tbsp. cocoa powder
6   packets artificial sweetener
     (not aspartame)
1   tsp. vanilla extract
1   extra large egg
¼   c. canned evaporated nonfat milk
¼   c. chopped pecans
     Nonstick cooking spray

BLUE-RIBBON BROWNIE TRIFLE
Contributed by Kay Smith, Roscoe, Texas

Break *Blue-Ribbon Brownies* into pieces; layer ½ of pieces in bottom of clear dish; set aside. In separate bowls, prepare vanilla and chocolate puddings, each according to package directions. Use ½ of chocolate pudding to layer over brownies in dish; use ½ of vanilla pudding to layer over chocolate. Repeat layers beginning with remaining brownie pieces. Top with whipped topping and pecans. Serves 12.
Exchanges: 1 bread, ¾ milk, 1 fat

BLUE-RIBBON BROWNIES
Contributed by Kay Smith, Roscoe, Texas

Preheat oven to 350° F. In medium bowl, combine baking mix, yogurt, cocoa powder, 4 packets sweetener, vanilla extract, egg and evaporated milk; mix well and pour into 13x9-inch baking dish coated with cooking spray. Top with chopped pecans; bake 15 minutes. Allow to cool 10 minutes; sprinkle remaining sweetener over top. Serves 8.
Exchanges: 1 bread, ¼ milk, ½ fat

Tip: Bake two batches and freeze one for later to use in the scrumptious *Blue-Ribbon Brownie Trifle!*

CHOCOLATE ECLAIR DESSERT

Contributed by Lisa Cramer, Houston, Texas

24	low-fat graham crackers
2	.8 oz. boxes sugar-free vanilla-flavored nonfat instant pudding
4 ½	c. nonfat milk, divided
4 ½	c. fat-free whipped topping
1	1.4 oz. box sugar-free chocolate-flavored nonfat instant pudding

Line bottom of a 13x9-inch baking dish with 8 graham crackers; set aside. In medium bowl, combine vanilla pudding mix with 3 cups milk; let sit 2 minutes. Gently fold in fat-free whipped topping; pour half over graham crackers in dish. Top with another 8 crackers. Pour remaining pudding over crackers. Top with last 8 crackers. Mix chocolate pudding mix with 1 ½ cups of milk; pour over top layer of graham crackers. Crumble remaining graham crackers over top; refrigerate 15 to 30 minutes. Serves 18.

Exchanges: 1 bread, ½ milk

FLUFFY FRUIT DESSERT

Contributed by Martha Rogers, Houston, Texas

4	low-fat graham crackers, broken into 16 pieces
8	oz. fat-free cream cheese
8	oz. artificially sweetened lemon-flavored nonfat yogurt
1	8-oz. can mandarin oranges, canned in water, drained
1	8-oz. can pineapple chunks in juice, drained
1	banana, cut in chunks
3	c. fat-free whipped topping

Line 13x9-inch baking dish with graham-cracker pieces. Beat together cream cheese and yogurt in medium bowl until smooth. Stir in fruits; then gently fold in whipped topping. Pour over graham crackers; refrigerate at least 3 hours. Serves 12.

Exchanges: ½ meat, ½ fruit

- 4 apples, peeled and sliced
- 1 tbsp. sugar
- ½ tsp. cinnamon, divided
- ¼ c. quick-cooking oats
- 1 tbsp. brown sugar
- 2 ½ tbsp. flour
- 1 tbsp. reduced-fat margarine, melted

- 3 apples, chopped
- 1 c. whole grapes
- 1 c. mandarin oranges
- ¼ c. raisins
- 1 c. walnuts or pecans
- 1 8-oz. container artificially sweetened plain nonfat yogurt

FRUIT CRISP

Contributed by Kay Smith, Roscoe, Texas

Preheat oven to 375° F. Place apple slices in 9-inch pie plate; set aside. In small bowl, combine sugar and ¼ teaspoon cinnamon; sprinkle over apples and toss gently to coat. Cover and bake 25 minutes; remove from oven and set aside. In separate bowl, combine oats, brown sugar, flour, margarine and remaining cinnamon; sprinkle over apples and return to oven. Bake uncovered 15 to 20 minutes or until fruit is tender. Serves 6.

Exchanges: 1 fruit

Tip: For a tasty variety, substitute pears or peaches for the apples!

FRUIT SALAD

Contributed by Daisy O. Mixon, Columbia, South Carolina

Combine fruits and nuts in large bowl; add yogurt and stir to coat. Refrigerate 2 hours. Serves 8.

Exchanges: 1 fruit, 2 fats

OATMEAL AND PECAN BARS

Contributed by Curtis Reuben, New Orleans, Louisiana

Preheat oven to 375° F. Combine oats, flour, sugar and baking soda in large bowl; mix well. Pour melted margarine over oatmeal mixture, blending together with hands until evenly moistened. Layer half the mixture over the bottom of 9x13-inch baking pan coated with cooking spray; top with thin layer of chopped pecans. Cover with remaining oat mixture and pat into place. Bake 20 minutes on middle shelf in oven; cool completely before cutting into 24 bars. Store in an airtight container with wax paper between layers. Serves 24.

Exchanges: 1 bread, 1½ fats

Tip: This recipe is kid friendly! For best results, use your hands to mix the ingredients.

2 c. quick-cooking oats
1 c. unbleached flour
1 c. firmly packed dark brown sugar
1 tsp. baking soda
½ c. unsalted margarine, melted
1 c. pecan halves, chopped
   Nonstick cooking spray

OATMEAL DELIGHT

Contributed by Jennifer Nelson, Little Rock, Mississippi

Combine oats, water, raisins and apple in a medium-sized, microwave-safe bowl. Microwave on high 2½ minutes or until thickened. Stir in peanut butter and season to taste with cinnamon, salt and sweetener. Allow to sit 2 minutes before serving. Serves 1.

Exchanges: 1½ breads, 1½ fruits, 1 fat

Tip: You can substitute an equal amount of nonfat milk for the water. (Add 1 milk exchange.)

⅓ c. quick-cooking oats
1 c. water
2 tbsp. raisins
½ apple, chopped
1 tsp. peanut butter
   Cinnamon to taste
   Salt to taste
   Artificial sweetener to taste
   (not aspartame)

1 20-oz. can pineapple chunks
   in juice, drained
1 8-oz. can crushed pineapple,
   drained
6 packets artificial sweetener
1 24-oz. container fat-free
   cottage cheese
3 c. fat-free whipped topping
2 1.4-oz. boxes sugar-free white-
   chocolate-flavored nonfat instant
   pudding
2 c. nonfat milk
¼ c. chopped pecans (optional)

1 32-oz. container artificially
   sweetened vanilla-flavored low-fat
   yogurt
4 8-oz. containers artificially
   sweetened banana-cream-pie-
   flavored low-fat yogurt
3 c. fat-free whipped topping
1 .3-oz. box sugar-free strawberry-
   banana-flavored gelatin
5 c. strawberries
2 bananas
2 c. Honey Bunches of Oats cereal,
   crushed

PINEAPPLE DREAM

Contributed by Joyce Luke, Meridian, Mississippi

In large bowl, combine both cans pineapple with 3 packets sweetener; set aside. In separate large bowl, mix together cottage cheese and remaining packets of sweetener; gently fold in whipped topping and set aside. In medium bowl, combine both pudding mixes with milk; fold into cottage-cheese mixture. Stir in pineapple; pour mixture into 9x13-inch baking dish and refrigerate at least 2 hours. Garnish with pecans if desired. Serves 15.
Exchanges: ½ meat, ½ bread, ¾ fruit

STRAWBERRY SURPRISE

Contributed by Lisa Cramer, Houston, Texas

Combine yogurts and fat-free whipped topping together in large bowl; stir in gelatin and blend well. Refrigerate several hours until ready to serve.

When ready to serve, remove from refrigerator and stir. Slice strawberries and bananas; divide evenly into serving bowls. Spoon yogurt mixture over fruit; sprinkle 1 tablespoon crushed cereal as topping over each serving. Serves 16.
Exchanges: ½ bread, ½ milk, ½ fruit

Tip: This is a fun dessert to experiment with! Try combining different flavors of low-fat, sugar-free yogurt, sugar-free gelatin and other fruits of choice.

To eliminate the bread exchange, leave off the cereal topping.

YOGURT SOFT-SERVE SURPRISE
Contributed by Ann Hykin, Clearwater, Florida

1 6-oz. container low-fat yogurt
6 oz. nonfat milk
1 c. berries (any kind, frozen or fresh)
2 packets artificial sweetener

Combine all ingredients in blender; blend until smooth. Pour into chilled ice-cream container; chill until soft-serve consistency. Serves 1.

Exchanges: 1½ milk, ½ fruit

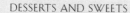

ENTRÉES

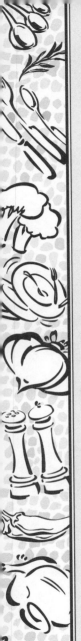

1 lb. lean ground beef
1 medium onion, chopped
1 10.7-oz. can low-fat cream of mushroom soup
1 10.7-oz. can low-fat cream of chicken soup
1 16-oz. jar picante sauce
8 oz. Velveeta Light processed cheese
12 tortillas, quartered

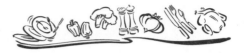

Entrées

BEEF AND VENISON

AUNT LOTTIE'S CROCK-POT ENCHILADAS

Contributed by Stacy Bowden, Gilmer, Texas

Brown ground beef and onion in skillet over medium heat. Drain and remove from skillet; set aside. Combine the mushroom and chicken soups with picante sauce in small bowl; mix well and set aside. Layer tortillas, browned meat and onions, soup mixture and cheese in Crock-Pot, repeating layers until all ingredients have been used. Cook on high 1 hour or until bubbly. Serves 8.

Exchanges: 3 meats, 1 ½ breads, 1 ½ fats

CABBAGE JAMBALAYA

Contributed by Judy Marshall, Gilmer, Texas

Cook ground beef in skillet over medium heat. Drain, rinse and return to skillet. Add onion, celery and bell pepper to skillet; sauté until tender. Stir in tomatoes, cabbage, rice and water; season to taste with garlic powder, salt and pepper. Cover and cook on low heat 45 minutes or until rice is done. Serves 8.

Exchanges: 2 meats, ½ bread, 1 vegetable

1   lb. lean ground beef
1   large onion, chopped
2   celery stalks, chopped
1   bell pepper, chopped
1   14.5-oz. can Rotel tomatoes
1   head green cabbage, chopped
½   c. white rice, uncooked
1   c. water
    Garlic powder to taste
    Salt and pepper to taste

CAJUN MEAT LOAF

Contributed by Johnny Lewis, San Leon, Texas

Preheat oven to 350° F. In small bowl, combine ½ cup ketchup and 1 tablespoon Pickapeppa sauce; stir well and set aside. In large bowl, combine ground round, onions, celery, bell pepper, garlic, remaining Pickapeppa sauce, Worcestershire sauce, remaining ketchup, milk, egg whites, bread crumbs, salt, and cayenne and black peppers; mix well. Shape into loaf and place in loaf pan; bake uncovered 25 minutes. Remove loaf; top with ketchup sauce and return to oven. Raise oven setting to 400° F and cook loaf 30 minutes more. Serves 10.

Exchanges: 3 meats, ½ bread

2   lbs. ground round
1   c. ketchup, divided
4   tbsp. Pickapeppa sauce (or your
    favorite steak sauce), divided
¾   c. finely chopped onion
¼   c. finely chopped green onion tops
½   c. finely chopped celery
½   c. finely chopped bell pepper
2   tsp. minced garlic
1   tbsp. Worcestershire sauce
½   c. nonfat milk
3   egg whites
1   c. bread crumbs
1   tsp. salt
½   tsp. cayenne pepper
1   tsp. black pepper

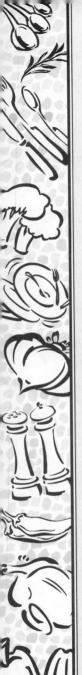

2 lbs. lean beef or venison, cut into
   bite-sized chunks
2 c. hot water
1 medium-sized brown onion, sliced
1 large bay leaf
1 tsp. Worcestershire sauce
1 tsp. sugar
¼ tsp. pepper
⅛ tsp. garlic powder
1 dash ground cloves
6 carrots, peeled and thinly sliced
4 potatoes, peeled and each cut into
   8 pieces
4 stalks celery, quartered lengthwise
1 lb. small white onions
¼ c. flour
⅓ c. cold water

EASY BEEF OR VENISON STEW
Contributed by Ann Hornbeak, Houston, Texas

Combine beef or venison, water, brown onion, bay leaf, Worcestershire sauce, sugar, pepper, garlic powder and cloves in microwave-safe dish. Cover and microwave on high 5 minutes; change power to 50 percent and continue cooking 40 minutes, stirring often to prevent sticking. Remove bay leaf and discard. Add carrots, potatoes, celery and white onions to meat mixture; cover and cook at 50 percent power 35 to 45 minutes more, stirring often. In small bowl, combine flour and cold water; blend well and stir into stew. Return to microwave; cook on high 3 to 4 minutes, stirring once or twice. Let stand 10 minutes. Serves 8.
Exchanges: 3 meats, 1 bread, 2 vegetables

GREEN-PEPPER STEAK

Contributed by Sheri Jackson, Okmulgee, Oklahoma

In medium bowl, combine soy sauce, beef broth, cayenne pepper and cornstarch; stir well and set aside. Preheat large nonstick skillet over high heat; coat with cooking spray. Stir-fry beef strips until browned; remove from skillet and keep warm. Add onions, bell pepper and celery to skillet; stir-fry until tender-crisp (adding more cooking spray if needed to prevent sticking). Return beef to pan; stir in sauce and cook, stirring constantly, until thickened and bubbly. Cook and stir 2 minutes more; add tomatoes and continue cooking until just heated through. Divide mixture evenly into 4 servings, each over ⅔ cup rice. Serves 4.

Exchanges: 4 meats, 2 breads, 2 vegetables

Tip: For easier slicing, cut meat while it is partially frozen.

1 lb. boneless top sirloin, fat removed and cut into bite-sized strips
¼ c. soy sauce
¼ c. beef broth
⅛ tsp. cayenne pepper (or to taste)
1 tbsp. cornstarch
2 small onions, thinly sliced
1 bell pepper, cut into 1-in. strips
2 celery stalks, sliced diagonally
1 garlic clove, minced
2 tomatoes, cut into wedges
2⅔ c. cooked white rice
Nonstick cooking spray

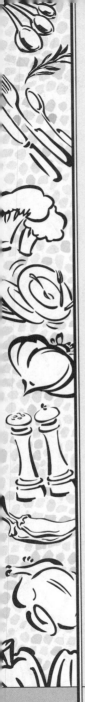

1 ½ lbs. lean ground beef
1 16-oz. can diced tomatoes
1 ½ tsp. ground cumin
¼ tsp. ground red pepper
¼ tsp. garlic powder
1 tsp. chili powder
1 tsp. black pepper
¼ tsp. salt
10 corn tortillas, cut into ¾ x 1-in. strips
2 c. fat-free cottage cheese
4 oz. part-skim mozzarella cheese
¼ c. egg substitute
½ c. chopped cilantro
2 c. shredded lettuce
1 c. chopped tomatoes
½ c. chopped green onions
Green or red salsa, if desired
Nonstick cooking spray

JAMIE'S MEXICAN LASAGNA

Contributed by Brenda Starry, Piedmont, Oklahoma

Preheat oven to 350° F. Preheat medium skillet; coat with cooking spray. Brown meat over medium heat; drain, rinse and return to skillet. Add tomatoes, cumin, red pepper, garlic powder, chili powder, black pepper and salt; heat thoroughly, stirring occasionally.

Use half the tortilla strips to layer bottom and sides of 9x13-inch baking dish coated with cooking spray. Pour beef mixture over tortillas in dish; layer remaining tortillas over meat. In medium bowl, combine cottage cheese, mozzarella, egg substitute and cilantro; mix well. Spoon over tortillas. Bake 30 minutes. Garnish with lettuce, tomatoes, green onions and salsa. Serves 10.

Exchanges: 3 meats, 1 bread, ½ vegetable

LIGHT MEXICAN MANICOTTI

Contributed by Julie Blackburn, Camden, Tennessee

In medium bowl, combine beef, beans, chili powder and oregano; mix well. Stuff mixture into manicotti shells; arrange in 13x9-inch baking dish coated with cooking spray. In small bowl, combine water and picante sauce; stir and pour over shells. Cover and refrigerate overnight.

Remove dish from refrigerator 30 minutes before baking. Preheat oven to 350° F. Bake covered 1 hour; uncover and spoon sour cream over top. Sprinkle with cheese, onions, tomatoes and jalapeños, if desired. Bake 5 to 10 minutes more or until cheese is melted. Serves 12.

Exchanges: 1 meat, 1 ½ breads, 1 fat

....
Tip: You can serve this dish with 1 cup fresh green salad and 2 tablespoons fat-free dressing. (Add 1 vegetable exchange.)
....

1   lb. lean ground beef
1   16-oz. can fat-free refried beans
2 ½   tsp. chili powder
1 ½   tsp. oregano
1   8-oz. pkg. manicotti pasta shells
2 ½   c. water
1   16-oz. jar picante sauce
2   c. low-fat sour cream
1   c. fat-free cheddar cheese
¼   c. sliced green onions
½   c. chopped tomatoes
¼   c. sliced jalapeño peppers (optional)
Nonstick cooking spray

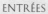

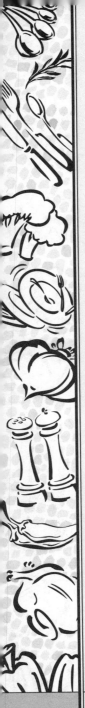

1   lb. ground venison
1   c. chopped onions
1   2 ½-oz. pkg. taco seasoning mix
1   10-oz. pkg. frozen chopped
    spinach, thawed and well drained
1   c. cottage cheese, drained
1   16-oz. box hot roll mix
1   egg, beaten with 1 tsp. water
    Nonstick cooking spray

MEXICAN-STYLE VENISON TORTE

Contributed by Terri Reed, Monroe, Washington

Preheat oven to 350° F. Lightly coat bottom and sides of 8-inch springform pan with cooking spray; set aside. Use medium nonstick skillet to cook venison (or beef) and onions over medium heat for 6 to 8 minutes or until meat is no longer pink, stirring occasionally. Drain; stir in seasoning mix and cook 2 minutes more, stirring frequently. Remove from heat; set aside. In small bowl, combine spinach and cottage cheese; set aside.

Prepare hot roll mix as directed on package. Divide dough in half and roll into 12-inch circle on lightly floured surface. Fit circle into prepared pan, pressing dough over bottom and up sides. Spoon meat mixture evenly into dough-lined pan; top with spinach mixture. Roll remaining dough into 9-inch circle on lightly floured surface; place over top and tuck edges of dough around inside of pan. Cut several 1-inch slits in top of dough to vent. Brush top of torte with beaten egg mixture; bake 45 to 50 minutes or until deep-golden brown. Let stand 10 minutes before removing sides of pan. Cut into 8 wedges. Serves 8.

Exchanges: 2 meats, 3 breads, ½ vegetable, 1 fat

Tip: This recipe also works great with lean ground beef instead of venison!

SHEPHERD'S PIE

Contributed by June Chapko, San Antonio, Texas

Preheat oven to 350° F. In large skillet over medium-high heat, cook ground beef, onion, salt and pepper until meat is browned. Add carrots and mushrooms; mix gently and reduce heat to simmer. In saucepan, prepare gravy mix according to package directions; slowly stir into meat mixture to distribute evenly. Pour into ungreased 2½-quart baking dish; set aside. Prepare mashed potatoes according to package directions, omitting milk and using only water. Spoon potatoes to form a ring around perimeter of meat; sprinkle cheese over top of potatoes and place in oven just long enough to melt cheese (approximately 3 minutes). Serves 4.
Exchanges: 4 meats, 2 breads, 2 vegetables, ½ milk

1 lb. lean ground beef
(or ground sirloin)
1 small onion, chopped
Salt and pepper to taste
1 14.5-oz. can sliced carrots, drained
1 2-oz. can sliced mushrooms, drained
4 tbsp. brown gravy mix
2 c. instant mashed potato flakes
4 oz. low-fat cheddar cheese

SPAGHETTI DELUXE

Contributed by Elizabeth Price, Gaffney, South Carolina

Preheat oven to 350° F. Prepare spaghetti according to package directions; drain and set aside. In medium bowl, blend milk and egg; add spaghetti and toss to coat. Spread spaghetti mixture in 10x15-inch baking dish coated with cooking spray; set aside. In large skillet, cook beef, onion and bell pepper until beef is no longer pink; drain and add tomato sauce, salt and pepper. Simmer 5 minutes; spoon over spaghetti. Top with mushrooms and cheese. Bake 20 minutes. Let stand 5 minutes before cutting. Serves 8.
Exchanges: 3 meats, ½ vegetable, 1 fat

½ lb. lean ground beef
7 oz. uncooked spaghetti
½ c. nonfat milk
1 egg, beaten
1 medium onion, chopped
1 medium bell pepper, chopped
1 15-oz. can tomato sauce
1 tsp. salt
¼ tsp. pepper
2 c. mushrooms, sliced
2 c. shredded part-skim mozzarella cheese
Nonstick cooking spray

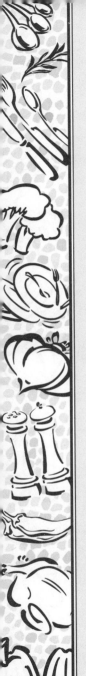

1 ½ lbs. round steak, tenderized and cut
        into 6 equal-sized pieces
1   onion, chopped
2   cloves garlic, minced
2   28-oz. cans diced tomatoes
1   4-oz. can chopped green chiles
1   tsp. salt, divided
¼   c. flour
¼   tsp. pepper
     Nonstick cooking spray

1   lb. lean ground beef
⅔   c. chopped onion or celery (optional)
1   tbsp. mustard
2   tbsp. ketchup
½   tsp. salt
⅛   tsp. pepper
1   10.7-oz. can low-fat cream of
        chicken soup
6   hamburger buns
     Nonstick cooking spray

SPICY SWISS STEAK

Contributed by Martha Rogers, Houston, Texas

Preheat oven to 325° F. Sauté onion and garlic in skillet coated with cooking spray until onion is opaque in color. Add tomatoes, green chiles and 1 teaspoon salt. Simmer uncovered 20 to 25 minutes or until slightly thickened.

In shallow bowl, combine flour, remaining salt and pepper; mix well. Dredge meat in flour mixture; brown in preheated skillet coated with cooking spray. When browned on both sides, transfer meat to 9x13-inch baking dish; pour half of tomato mixture over meat, reserving remainder. Cover and bake 1 hour or until meat is tender. Heat reserved sauce; pour over steak prior to serving. Serves 8.
Exchanges: 3 meats, 1 ½ vegetables

SPOONBURGERS BARBECUE

Contributed by Janet Kirkhart, Mount Orab, Ohio

In medium skillet coated with cooking spray, brown beef and onion or celery; drain and rinse with water. Return to pan and add mustard, ketchup, salt and pepper; stir well and allow to cook 1 to 2 minutes. Add soup and simmer 30 minutes. Spoon onto hamburger bun. Serves 6.
Exchanges: 3 meats, 2 breads

ENTRÉES

Beef and Venison

STAY-SLIM LASAGNA

Contributed by Lisa Cramer, Houston, Texas

Preheat oven to 350° F. Brown beef, onion and garlic in preheated skillet over medium heat; add Italian dressing, basil, parsley, red pepper, water and tomato paste, and salt and pepper to taste. Simmer 10 minutes; stir in mushrooms. In separate saucepan, use water to steam spinach, stirring occasionally until spinach is wilted. Drain and mash out excess liquid, using wire strainer. Return to saucepan and add ¼ teaspoon black pepper, if desired. Stir in all of the ricotta and ½ of the mozzarella. Boil 6 lasagna noodles according to package directions (omitting salt and fat), until tender; drain. Line bottom of 9x9-inch or 7x11-inch baking dish with 3 lasagna noodles; then layer remaining ingredients in following order: ½ meat mixture, all of spinach-cheese mixture, remaining lasagna noodles and remaining meat mixture. Bake 30 minutes. Top with remaining mozzarella prior to serving. Serves 6.

Exchanges: 3 meats, 1 bread, 1½ vegetables, ½ fat

Tip: You can substitute a 10-ounce package of frozen chopped spinach for the fresh spinach leaves. Simply thaw and use a wire strainer to drain excess water before using.

½ lb. lean ground beef or turkey
½ c. chopped onion
1 tsp. chopped garlic
½ tsp. Italian salad dressing
½ tsp. basil
1 tbsp. dried parsley
¼ tsp. crushed red pepper
½ c. water
6 oz. tomato paste
Salt and pepper to taste
1 c. sliced mushrooms
2 c. spinach leaves
¼ tsp. black pepper (optional)
6 oz. part-skim ricotta cheese
6 oz. shredded mozzarella cheese, divided
6 lasagna noodles

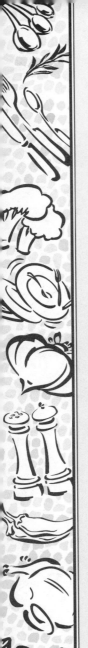

3 lbs. extra-lean ground beef
1 lb. pinto beans, rinsed
1 tbsp. seasoned salt
4 ½ tbsp. chili powder, divided
2 tsp. cumin, divided
2 tsp. paprika, divided
5 qts. plus 2 c. water
1 c. chopped onion
1 8-oz. can tomato sauce
6 garlic cloves, chopped
1 tsp. oregano
1 tbsp. salt
Salt and pepper to taste
Nonstick cooking spray

1 ½ lbs. lean ground beef or turkey
½ c. minced onion, divided
¼ c. egg substitute
¼ c. nonfat milk
2 slices whole-grain bread, cubed
½ tsp. salt
½ tsp. pepper
1 packet artificial sweetener
(not aspartame)
½ tsp. allspice
½ tsp. nutmeg
4 tbsp. fat-free brown gravy mix
¼ c. evaporated nonfat milk
Parsley for garnish, chopped
Nonstick cooking spray

ENTRÉES

Beef and Venison

SUPERB CHILI AND BEANS

Contributed by Johnny Lewis, San Leon, Texas

Combine pinto beans, seasoned salt, 1 tablespoon chili powder, 1 teaspoon cumin, 1 teaspoon paprika and 5 quarts water into 1 ½-gallon cooking pot. Bring to rolling boil; reduce heat and boil gently 1 ½ hours.

Preheat large nonstick cooking pot coated with cooking spray. Cook beef and onion over medium heat until meat is gray in color; drain excess liquid. Stir in tomato sauce, 2 cups water, 3 ½ tablespoons chili powder, 1 teaspoon cumin, garlic, 1 teaspoon oregano, 1 teaspoon paprika and 1 tablespoon salt. Simmer uncovered 1 hour and 15 minutes.

Meantime, taste pinto beans for seasoning; add salt and pepper, if desired, and continue to gently boil 1 ½ hours more. Add beans to cooked chili and cook 30 minutes more on low heat, stirring often. Serves 20.

Exchanges: 2 meats, 1 bread

SWEDISH MEATBALLS

Contributed by Margaret Anderson, Houston, Texas

Preheat skillet coated with cooking spray; add ¼ cup onion and sauté until onion is just golden; remove from heat. In large mixing bowl, combine egg substitute, milk and bread cubes; let stand 5 minutes. Add salt, pepper, sweetener, allspice, nutmeg, meat and sautéed onion; blend well and shape into small balls (about ½ to ¾ inch in diameter). Brown several meatballs at a time in skillet used to sauté onion; turn meatballs until browned on all sides. Remove and place in warm casserole dish; repeat until all meatballs are done. Make gravy according to package directions; set aside. Brown remaining minced onion; add to gravy and pour over meatballs. Heat until warm; stir in evaporated milk and top with chopped parsley. Serves 6.

Exchanges: 3 meats, ½ bread

TAMALE PIE

Contributed by Sheri Jackson, Okmulgee, Oklahoma

Preheat oven to 375° F. Brown ground beef, onion and bell pepper in skillet coated with cooking spray; drain. Stir in tomato sauce, tomatoes, corn, olives, garlic, sugar, ½ teaspoon salt, 2 teaspoons chili powder and dash black pepper. Bring mixture to boil; simmer uncovered 20 minutes or until thickened. Stir in cheese until melted; remove from heat and set aside. Combine cornmeal, remaining salt and chili powder, and water in saucepan; cook over medium-high heat, stirring constantly until thickened. Stir in margarine; mix well. Spread half of mixture over bottom of a 12x8-inch baking dish; add meat filling and spoon remaining cornmeal mixture over top. Bake 45 minutes. Serves 6.

Exchanges: 4 meats, 1½ breads, 1½ vegetables, 1 fat

Tip: Top this tasty dish with ½ cup reduced-fat cheddar cheese prior to serving, if desired. (Add ½ fat exchange.)

- 1 lb. lean ground beef
- 1 c. chopped onion
- 1 bell pepper, chopped
- 1 15-oz. can tomato sauce
- 1 28-oz. can diced tomatoes
- 1 17-oz. can corn, drained
- ½ c. olives, pitted and sliced
- 1 garlic clove, minced
- 1 tbsp. sugar
- 1 tsp. salt, divided
- 2½ tsp. chili powder, divided
  Dash black pepper
- 1 c. shredded low-fat cheddar cheese
- ¾ c. yellow cornmeal
- 2 c. cold water
- 1 tbsp. reduced-fat margarine
  Nonstick cooking spray

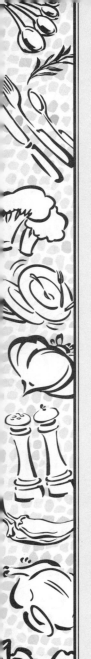

8 oz. lean ground beef

12 6-in. thin corn tortillas

1 medium onion, chopped

1 2 ½-oz. pkg. taco seasoning mix

1 15-oz. can pinto beans, drained
and rinsed

8 oz. Velveeta Light processed cheese,
sliced

1 10.7-oz. can reduced-fat cream of
chicken soup

1 14.5-oz. can Rotel tomatoes
Nonstick cooking spray

2 lbs. lean ground venison, crumbled

1 16-oz. can refried beans

1 15-oz. can tomato sauce

1 c. chopped onion

1 c. shredded cheddar cheese

1 4-oz. can chopped green chiles,
drained

1 ½ tsp. chili powder

½ tsp. ground cumin

½ tsp. ground pepper

¼ tsp. ground cloves

16 10-in. flour tortillas

TEAGUE TORTILLA BAKE
Contributed by Judy Marshall, Gilmer, Texas

Preheat oven to 350° F. Brown ground beef and onion in skillet coated with cooking spray; add taco seasoning and mix well. Layer 9x13-inch baking dish coated with cooking spray in following order: 6 tortillas, ½ of meat mixture, ½ of beans and ½ of cheese. Repeat layers; set aside. In small bowl, combine soup and tomatoes; mix well and pour over top of tortillas. Bake 30 minutes or until bubbly. Serves 8.
Exchanges: 2 meats, 3 breads, ½ vegetable, ½ fat

VENISON BURRITOS
Contributed by Terri Reed, Monroe, Washington

Preheat oven to 350° F. Use medium heat to cook meat in skillet 10 to 12 minutes or until no longer pink, stirring occasionally. Drain; stir in refried beans, tomato sauce, onion, cheese, chiles, chili powder, cumin, pepper and cloves. Reduce heat to medium low; cook 30 to 40 minutes more or until flavors are blended, stirring occasionally. Warm tortillas as directed on package. Place ½ cup meat mixture in center of each tortilla; fold bottom half of tortilla over filling and then fold over sides and top. Place burritos seam-side down on baking sheet; bake 8 to 10 minutes or until hot. Serve with desired toppings (e.g., salsa, pico de gallo or chopped onion). Serves 16.
Exchanges: 1 ½ meats, 2 ½ breads, ½ vegetable, 2 ½ fats

Tip: You can substitute the same amount of lean ground beef for the venison, if desired.

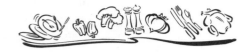

FISH AND SEAFOOD

BAKED STUFFED FISH
Contributed by Janet Bayless, Clinton, Tennessee

Preheat oven to 400° F. Sauté onion until tender in large skillet coated with cooking spray. Add crumbled bread, basil and pepper; mix well. Layer stuffing mixture over bottom of 8x8-inch baking dish coated with cooking spray; arrange fillets over stuffing. Melt margarine and drizzle over fish; garnish with paprika. Bake 15 to 20 minutes or until fish flakes easily with fork. Serves 4.
Exchanges: 1 ½ meats, ½ bread, ¼ fat

4	2-oz. portions of whitefish fillets
½	c. chopped onion
4	slices reduced-calorie bread, crumbled
1	tsp. basil
⅛	tsp. black pepper
3	tsp. reduced-calorie margarine
½	tsp. paprika
	Butter-flavored nonstick cooking spray

> **Tip:** Day-old or slightly dry bread makes for great homemade bread crumbs!

EXTRAORDINARY BAKED SALMON
Contributed by Carol Moore, Meridian, Mississippi

Preheat oven to 450° F. In oven, preheat baking dish drizzled with olive oil. Place fillets skin-side down on flat surface; rub with lemon juice. Sprinkle with seasonings in following order: rosemary, paprika, adobo, black pepper and salt. Lightly drizzle with honey; sprinkle with pecans and seal with generous coating of cooking spray. Place fillets skin-side down in preheated baking dish; bake 10 to 15 minutes or until fillets flake easily with fork. Serves 6.
Exchanges: 3 meats, ½ fat

6	4-oz. salmon fillets, each 1 in. thick
1	tbsp. olive oil
	Splash lemon juice
	(enough to moisten each fillet)
	Fresh rosemary to taste
	Paprika to taste
	Adobo seasoning to taste
	Black pepper to taste
	Salt to taste
	Honey to taste
¼	c. finely chopped pecans
	Nonstick cooking spray

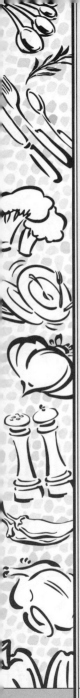

1 lb. cooked shrimp, peeled and deveined

½ c. fat-free chicken broth

1 medium onion, chopped

½ c. minced green bell pepper

1 garlic clove, minced

1 tsp. salt

Dash pepper

⅛ tsp. paprika

1 tsp. chili powder

2 to 3 dashes Tabasco sauce

1 tsp. Filé brand gumbo seasoning

2 14½-oz. cans Cajun-style
stewed tomatoes

2⅔ c. cooked white rice

QUICK AND EASY SHRIMP CREOLE
Contributed by Peggy Grooms, Sherman, Texas

Combine broth, onion, green pepper and garlic in medium saucepan; sauté until tender-crisp. Add salt, pepper, paprika, chili powder, Tabasco sauce, gumbo seasoning and stewed tomatoes; bring to a boil and add shrimp. Reduce heat; simmer 15 minutes. Serve over ⅔ cup cooked rice. Serves 4.

Exchanges: 2 meats, 2 breads, 2½ vegetables

SEAFOOD PRIMAVERA

Contributed by Barbara Bartlett, Kensington, Maryland

Cook linguine according to package directions, omitting salt and fat; drain well and set aside in very large bowl (keep warm). Cook onions in oil in large skillet over medium-high heat until soft. Add carrots, zucchini, squash, bell pepper, snow peas, mushrooms and garlic; reduce heat to low. Cover and simmer until vegetables are tender; remove from skillet and set aside. Use same skillet to cook shrimp and scallops over medium-low heat until opaque; then remove from pan and reserve liquid. In medium bowl, combine flour, bouillon, water and milk; stir until flour is completely dissolved. Pour into skillet and bring to slow boil, stirring constantly until thickened. Reduce heat to low; add cheese and stir until smooth. Add vegetable mixture, shrimp, scallops and crabmeat; heat through. Add lemon juice, parsley, basil, oregano and black pepper; pour mixture over linguine; toss gently to coat. Serves 6.

Exchanges: 2½ meats, 2 breads, 1 vegetable, ½ fat

½ lb. shrimp, peeled and deveined
½ lb. scallops
⅔ c. flaked crabmeat
8 oz. linguine
1 medium onion, chopped
4 green onions, chopped
1 tbsp. olive oil
3 carrots, julienne
1 small zucchini, julienne
1 small yellow squash, julienne
1 small red bell pepper, julienne
3 oz. snow peas
⅓ c. sliced mushrooms
3 garlic cloves, minced
2 tbsp. flour
1 chicken bouillon cube
1 c. water
1 c. milk
½ c. Parmesan cheese
2 tbsp. lemon juice
2 tbsp. fresh parsley
(or 1½ tbsp. dried)
¼ tsp. dried basil
¼ tsp. dried oregano
Black pepper to taste

ENTRÉES

Fish and Seafood

1 lb. shrimp, peeled and deveined

3 tbsp. reduced-calorie margarine

1 c. combined chopped onion, celery, green bell pepper and garlic (can omit any)

1 10.7-oz. can low-fat cream of celery soup

10 slices bread, lightly toasted and cut into squares

2 tbsp. bread crumbs

2 6-oz. cans tuna

2 tsp. prepared green-chile dip

4 6-in. whole-wheat tortillas

½ c. shredded fat-free cheddar cheese

SHRIMP CASSEROLE

Contributed by Inez Boudreaux, Scott, Louisiana

Preheat oven to 350° F. Use skillet and margarine to sauté vegetables until tender; add shrimp and cook until opaque. Add soup and stir well; simmer 10 minutes. Add bread squares; season to taste and mix well. Pour into 2-quart baking dish; sprinkle top with bread crumbs. Bake uncovered 20 minutes or until heated through. Serves 4.

Exchanges: 2 meats, 3 breads, 1 fat

TUNA BURRITO

Contributed by Favi Sotelo, Artesia, New Mexico

In small bowl, combine tuna and chile dip; mix well. Warm tortillas in microwave or on stove top; cover with tuna mixture and sprinkle each with 2 tablespoons cheese. Serves 4.

Exchanges: 3 meats, 2½ meats, 2½ breads, 1 fat

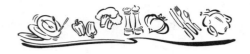

MEATLESS MEALS

CHEESE ENCHILADAS
Contributed by Judy Marshall, Gilmer, Texas

Preheat oven to 325° F. Heat soup, chiles, milk and Velveeta over low heat, stirring frequently until melted. Pour ½ cup cheese sauce into bottom of 7x11-inch baking dish coated with cooking spray. Place 1 ounce grated cheese in center of each tortilla and roll up (or ½ ounce in each if using corn tortillas). Place seamside down into baking dish; pour remaining sauce over tortillas. Garnish with fresh cilantro, if desired. Bake 20 to 25 minutes. Serves 5.

Exchanges: 2 meat, 1½ bread, 1½ fat

....

Tip: You can make meat and cheese enchiladas by using 10 ounces taco meat prepared with lean ground beef or 10 ounces fajita-style cooked chicken per serving. (Add 2 meat exchanges.)

....

5 8-in. flour tortillas
   (or 10 6-in. thin corn tortillas)
1 10.7-oz. can reduced-fat cream of
   chicken soup
1 4.5 oz. can chopped green chiles
6 oz. evaporated nonfat milk
8 oz. Velveeta Light processed cheese
5 oz. cheddar cheese, grated
   Fresh cilantro (optional)
   Nonstick cooking spray

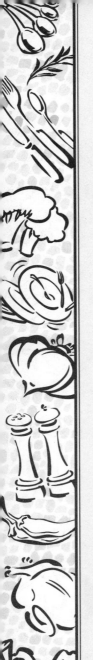

6 lasagna noodles
3 c. chopped and cooked broccoli
¼ c. nonfat Parmesan cheese
½ c. nonfat ricotta cheese
½ c. nonfat cottage cheese
2 c. spaghetti sauce, divided
Nonstick cooking spray

1 2-oz. slice French bread
1½ tbsp. pizza sauce
2 oz. part-skim mozzarella cheese
Choice of onions, mushrooms,
bell pepper or zucchini, sliced thin

1 12-oz. can green enchilada sauce
4 low-fat flour tortillas
1 c. grated low-fat cheddar cheese,
divided
½ c. fat-free sour cream
Fresh cilantro, chopped (optional)
Nonstick cooking spray

BROCCOLI LASAGNA ROLLS
Contributed by Patti McCoy, Fort Lupton, Colorado

Preheat oven to 350° F. Cook lasagna noodles according to package directions, omitting salt and fat. In medium bowl, mix broccoli and Parmesan, ricotta and cottage cheeses. Spread filling over lasagna; carefully roll up and arrange in 7x11-inch baking dish coated with cooking spray. Cover with spaghetti sauce and bake 20 minutes. Serves 6.
Exchanges: 1 meat, 3 vegetables, 1 fat

FRENCH BREAD VEGETABLE PIZZA
Contributed by Johnny Lewis, San Leon, Texas

Preheat oven to 375° F. Top bread with pizza sauce, cheese and vegetables. Bake until cheese melts, approximately 15 minutes. Serves 1.
Exchanges: 2 meats, 2 breads, ½ vegetable, 1 fat

Tip: You can substitute a 2-ounce bagel or English muffin for the French bread without altering the exchanges.

GREEN ENCHILADAS
Contributed by Judy Marshall, Gilmer, Texas

Preheat oven to 325° F. Warm enchilada sauce in nonstick skillet coated with cooking spray. Dip 1 tortilla in sauce to soften; remove from sauce and fill with ¼ cup cheese. Roll and place seam-side down in small baking dish coated with cooking spray. Repeat for remaining tortillas. Stir sour cream into remaining sauce; pour over enchiladas. Sprinkle with cilantro, if desired, and bake 20 to 25 minutes or until just heated through. Serves 4.
Exchanges: 1 meat, 1½ breads, 1 fat

GREEK SPAGHETTI

Contributed by Stephanie Cheves, Houston, Texas

Cook spaghetti according to package directions, omitting salt and fat; drain and set aside. Combine tomatoes, olives, basil, garlic powder, salt, pepper and olive oil in large saucepan; warm over medium heat. Add spaghetti to sauce; toss gently to coat and sprinkle with cheese. Serves 4.

Exchanges: 3 breads, 1 vegetable, 1 fat

8	oz. spaghetti
2	14.5-oz. cans diced tomatoes
1	4-oz. can sliced black olives, drained
1	tsp. dried basil
1/4	tsp. garlic powder
1/4	tsp. salt
1/8	tsp. pepper
2	tsp. olive oil
1/2	c. shredded Parmesan cheese

HEALTHY GREEK OMELET

Contributed by Cory Beckman, Vacaville, California

In nonstick skillet coated with cooking spray, sauté onion and spinach over medium heat until onions begin to soften and spinach is wilted. Distribute evenly in skillet and cover with egg substitute. When egg begins to set, loosen with spatula and turn over trying to keep intact. Sprinkle with feta cheese; salt and pepper to taste. Serves 1.

Exchanges: 2 meats, 3 vegetables, 1 fat

3	tbsp. chopped onion
1 1/2	c. torn fresh spinach leaves
1/2	c. Egg Beaters (or other 99% fat-free egg substitute)
1	oz. feta cheese
	Salt and pepper to taste
	Nonstick cooking spray

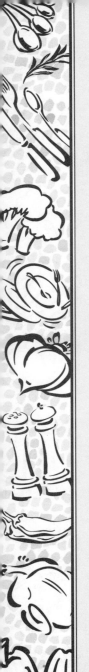

1 c. linguine
3 garlic cloves, thinly sliced
½ tsp. crushed red pepper
1 tbsp. olive oil
4 c. chopped fresh tomatoes
½ c. coarsely chopped fresh basil
2 tbsp. chopped fresh parsley
2 tbsp. red wine vinegar
½ tsp. salt
1 packet artificial sweetener
  (not aspartame)
  Fresh basil for garnish

1 6-in. whole-wheat pita
¼ c. tomato sauce
  Italian spices (oregano, basil or
  other seasonings as desired) to taste
  Salt and pepper to taste
2 oz. part-skim mozzarella cheese
1 c. sliced portobello mushrooms
2 small Roma tomatoes, sliced
1 tsp. grated Romano cheese
1 tsp. grated Parmesan cheese
  Butter-flavored nonstick
  cooking spray

LINGUINE WITH FRESH TOMATO SAUCE

Contributed by Carolyn Owen, Charlotte Court House, Virginia

Cook linguine according to package directions, omitting salt and fat; drain and set aside. In large skillet, sauté garlic and red pepper in oil over low heat. Add tomatoes, basil, parsley, vinegar, salt and sweetener; cook 3 to 5 minutes or until thickened. Toss linguine with sauce; garnish with fresh basil. Serves 2.

Exchanges: 2 breads, 2 vegetables, 1 ½ fats

Tip: You can garnish each serving with 2 tablespoons Parmesan cheese if you like. (Add ½ meat exchange.)

PITA PIZZA

Contributed by Shelly Wright, Colorado Springs, Colorado

Preheat oven to 400° F. Coat pita on both sides with cooking spray; bake 5 minutes or until crispy. Combine tomato sauce with Italian spices, salt and pepper to taste. Spread tomato mixture over pita; layer with mozzarella cheese (reserving about 1 tablespoon), mushrooms and tomatoes. Sprinkle top with Romano and Parmesan cheeses and remaining mozzarella. Garnish with more spices and place back in oven. Baked until cheese is bubbly. Serves 1.

Exchanges: 2½ meats, 2 breads, 2 vegetables

ROASTED RED PEPPER PASTA

Contributed by Stephanie Cheves, Houston, Texas

Preheat broiler. Coat bell peppers with cooking spray; arrange peppers and garlic on baking sheet lined with aluminum foil. Broil 5 minutes and turn; broil 5 minutes more and remove from broiler. Once cooled, slice open peppers and remove seeds and stems. Place peppers, garlic, olive oil and tomato puree in food processor or blender and blend until smooth. Add salt and pepper to taste. Toss pasta and sauce in large bowl. Serves 4.

Exchanges: 2 breads, 2 vegetables, ½ fat

4 medium red bell peppers
2 medium garlic cloves
2 tsp. olive oil
1 c. tomato puree
   Salt and pepper
4 c. cooked fusilli pasta, warm
   Olive oil nonstick cooking spray

SPINACH AND CHEESE MANICOTTI

Contributed by Connie Armstrong, Hattiesburg, Mississippi

Preheat oven to 350° F. Combine onion, spinach, bouillon, garlic powder, thyme, cottage cheese and egg whites in large bowl; mix well. Stir in ¼ cup Parmesan cheese and ½ cup mozzarella cheese. Scoop into manicotti; place single layer of filled shells in 9x13-inch baking dish. Sprinkle ½ cup mozzarella cheese over filled shells; pour half of spaghetti sauce evenly over top. Repeat with remaining mozzarella and sauce; top with remaining Parmesan cheese. Bake 30 minutes or until heated through. Serves 14.

Exchanges: 1½ meats, 1 bread, ½ fat

14 large manicotti pasta shells,
    cooked and cooled
½   c. finely chopped onion
1   10-oz. pkg. frozen chopped
    spinach, thawed
1   tbsp. reduced-sodium chicken bouillon
½   tsp. garlic powder
⅛   tsp. dried thyme leaves
1½ c. fat-free cottage cheese
3   egg whites
½   c. grated fat-free Parmesan cheese,
    divided
1½ c. part-skim mozzarella cheese,
    divided
26 oz. low-fat spaghetti sauce

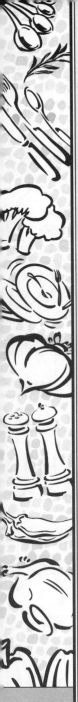

1   10-oz. pkg. frozen chopped
      spinach, thawed and drained

1   15-oz. pkg. low-fat ricotta cheese

1   c. grated Parmesan cheese, divided

1   c. low-fat plain yogurt

1   egg

¾ tsp. salt

¼ tsp. pepper

1   26-oz. jar low-fat spaghetti sauce

6   lasagna noodles

8   oz. part-skim mozzarella cheese,
      shredded and divided

1   c. water
      Nonstick cooking spray

SPINACH LASAGNA

Contributed by Janet Bayless, Clinton, Tennessee

Preheat oven to 375° F. Use hands to squeeze out as much excess liquid from spinach as possible. Combine spinach, ricotta cheese, ½ cup Parmesan cheese, yogurt, egg, salt and pepper in large bowl; mix thoroughly and set aside. Evenly spread ½ cup spaghetti sauce in 9x13-inch baking dish coated with cooking spray. Layer 3 lasagna noodles in bottom of dish, breaking last noodle to fit and fill space. Carefully spoon ½ of spinach-cheese mixture to create thin layer over noodles; sprinkle evenly with half of mozzarella cheese. Evenly spread half of remaining spaghetti sauce over cheese and repeat layers beginning with lasagna. Top with remaining Parmesan cheese.

Run a metal spatula or knife around edges of casserole, raising noodles slightly while carefully pouring water around the edges (don't worry if some of the water mixes with the spaghetti sauce). Cover tightly with foil and crimp edges. Bake 1 hour and 15 minutes; remove from oven and let stand 15 minutes covered. Serves 12.
Exchanges: 1 ½ meats, 2 vegetables, 1 ½ fats

ENTRÉES

Meatless Meals

STUFFED PASTA SHELLS

Contributed by Nancy Taylor, Houston, Texas

In a medium bowl, combine ricotta cheese, ½ of mozzarella cheese, egg, garlic, salt, pepper, parsley and other seasonings of choice; mix well and set aside. Pour ⅓ of spaghetti sauce into bottom of 9x13-inch baking dish. Use cheese mixture to stuff pasta shells; arrange stuffed shells in dish. Sprinkle with remaining mozzarella cheese and cover with remaining sauce. Bake uncovered 30 minutes or until sauce is bubbly. Serves 6.

Exchanges: 2 meats, 1 bread, 1 vegetable, 1 fat

1   16-oz. box large pasta shells, cooked until just tender and drained (do not overcook)

8   oz. part-skim ricotta cheese

8   oz. mozzarella cheese, shredded and divided

1   egg or egg substitute to equal 1 egg

½   tbsp. garlic

½   tbsp. salt

¼   tsp. pepper

½   tbsp. parsley

   Seasonings of choice to taste

1   26-oz. jar spaghetti sauce

VEGETABLE PESTO FETTUCCINE

Contributed by Tamara Taber, Orangeville, California

Place fettuccine in large bowl; toss with cooking spray and set aside. In small saucepan, whisk together pesto mix, vegetable broth, olive oil, garlic and black pepper; bring to a gentle boil, reduce heat and simmer 5 minutes. Place water, broccoli, carrots and squash in microwave-safe bowl; cover and cook on high 4 minutes. Stir Parmesan cheese and pine nuts into simmering pesto sauce; remove from heat. Add vegetables to fettuccine and top with pesto sauce; toss until well coated. Serves 1.

Exchanges: ½ meat, 2 breads, 2 vegetables, 2 fats

1   c. cooked fettuccine

1   ½-oz. pkg. pesto mix

1   14-oz. can vegetable broth

2   tsp. olive oil

1   garlic clove, minced

⅛   tsp. black pepper

2   tbsp. water

1   c. chopped broccoli

⅓   c. chopped carrots

½   c. chopped yellow squash

½   oz. Parmesan cheese, grated

1¼   tsp. dry-roasted pine nuts, chopped

   Nonstick cooking spray

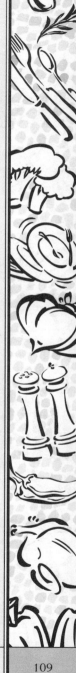

ENTRÉES

Meatless Meals

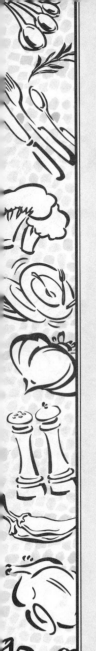

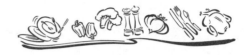

PORK

GOLDEN FRUITED HAM

Contributed by Kathi Reinecke, Riverview, Florida

2   lbs. extra-lean reduced-sodium ham, sliced and trimmed of fat
1   12-oz. jar apricot all-fruit spread
¼   c. firmly packed light brown sugar
2   tbsp. flour
1   tbsp. white wine vinegar
1   tbsp. Dijon mustard
½   tsp. ground ginger
⅛   tsp. ground cloves
1   15-oz. can apricot halves, drained and coarsely chopped
½   c. raisins
2   tbsp. cornstarch
2   tbsp. water

Trim fat from ham; place in 4-quart electric slow-cooker. In large bowl, combine all-fruit spread, brown sugar, flour, vinegar, mustard, ginger and cloves; stir well. Add apricots and raisins; stir well and pour over ham. Cover cooker with lid; cook on high setting 2 hours or until ham is thoroughly heated. Remove meat from cooker; set aside and keep warm. Pour cooking liquid into small saucepan; set aside. Combine cornstarch and water in small bowl; stir until smooth. Add to cooking liquid; bring to a boil and cook 1 minute or until thick, stirring constantly. Serve about ¼ cup sauce with each serving. Serves 6.

Exchanges: 3 meats, 4 breads, ½ fruit

PORK LO MEIN

Contributed by Stephanie Cheves, Houston, Texas

1   lb. pork tenderloin, cut into thin strips
¼   c. low-sodium soy sauce
3   cloves garlic
1   tsp. minced fresh gingerroot
¼   tsp. cayenne pepper
2   c. snow peas
1   medium red bell pepper, sliced
1   medium yellow bell pepper, sliced
1   medium onion, sliced
3   c. cooked spaghetti
½   c. chicken broth
    Nonstick cooking spray

Combine soy sauce, garlic, gingerroot and cayenne pepper in container; add pork and marinate 30 minutes. In preheated wok coated with cooking spray, stir-fry pork together with marinade over high heat 4 to 5 minutes or until meat is no longer pink. Add snow peas, peppers and onion; stir-fry until tender. Stir in cooked spaghetti and chicken broth. Cook about 1 minute more or until spaghetti is thoroughly coated. Serves 4.

Exchanges: 3 meats, 1½ breads, 2 vegetables

ENTRÉES

Pork

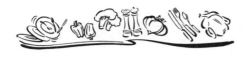

POULTRY

BALSAMIC CHICKEN WITH ROSEMARY

Contributed by Sheri Jackson, Okmulgee, Oklahoma

Place chicken in a shallow pan or plastic bag with seal; set aside. Combine oil, vinegar, lemon peel, lemon juice, rosemary, garlic, salt and pepper in small bowl; use wire whisk to blend. Pour marinade over chicken and refrigerate 1 to 3 hours. Grill or broil to liking. Serves 4.

Exchanges: 3½ meats, ½ fat

BARBECUE CHICKEN KABOBS

Contributed by Ann Ellis, Louisville, Mississippi

Combine chicken, shrimp (if desired), potatoes, squash, onions, tomatoes and peppers in large container with lid; set aside. In separate bowl, combine vinegar, oil, garlic salt, Worcestershire sauce, ketchup, mustard, salt, pepper and soy sauce. Stir well and pour marinade over chicken and vegetables; refrigerate 24 to 48 hours, stirring every 8 to 12 hours to coat.

Preheat grill to medium-high heat. Use skewers to create kabobs, alternating meat and vegetables and using 2 chunks chicken, 2 shrimp and 2 of each vegetable per skewer. Grill over medium-high heat 10 to 15 minutes or until meat is thoroughly cooked. Serves 4.

Exchanges: 3½ meats, 1 bread, 1 vegetable, ½ fat

- 4 cooked chicken breasts
- 1 tbsp. olive oil
- 4 tsp. balsamic vinegar
- 1 tsp. grated lemon peel
- 1 tsp. lemon juice
- ½ tsp. rosemary
- 1 garlic clove, minced or pressed
- ¼ tsp. salt
- ⅛ tsp. pepper

- 2 boneless, skinless chicken breasts, cubed
- 8 large shrimp (optional)
- 8 small new potatoes, cooked until almost done
- 2 yellow squash, cut into chunks
- 2 onions, cut into chunks
- 8 cherry tomatoes
- 2 bell peppers, cut into 2-in. pieces
- ⅓ c. red wine vinegar
- 2 tsp. vegetable oil
- ¼ tsp. garlic salt
- 1 tsp. Worcestershire sauce
- ¼ c. ketchup
- 1 tsp. prepared mustard
- 1 tsp. salt
- ¼ tsp. black pepper
- 2 tsp. low-sodium soy sauce

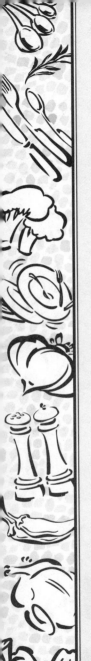

1 c. diced chicken breast

1 c. diced cooked ham

2 c. brown rice

2 garlic cloves, minced or pressed

½ c. diced onion

½ c. diced bell pepper

2 tbsp. olive oil

6 skinless chicken breasts

2 c. chopped onion

2 15-oz. cans corn

1 28-oz. can crushed tomatoes

1 12-oz. jar chili sauce

1 14-oz. can chicken broth

¼ c. Worcestershire sauce

2 tbsp. vinegar

2 tsp. dry mustard

½ tsp. salt

½ tsp. pepper

½ tsp. pepper sauce

1 c. instant rice, uncooked

BROWN RICE JAMBALAYA

Contributed by Eloria Phipps, New Orleans, Louisiana

Cook rice according to package directions. In nonstick skillet, use oil to sauté garlic, onion, bell pepper, chicken and ham over medium heat until juice from chicken runs clear and vegetables are tender. Salt and pepper to taste and serve over ¼ cup rice. Serves 8.

Exchanges: 1 ½ meats, 2 ½ breads, ½ vegetable, 1 fat

Tip: Try Mrs. Dash seasoning instead of salt to add some great flavor while reducing your sodium intake!

BRUNSWICK CROCK-POT STEW

Contributed by Joe Ann Winkler, Overland Park, Kansas

Layer all ingredients *in order* in 4-quart Crock-Pot set to high. Cook 4 hours; remove chicken (and pork, if desired) and allow to cool to touch. Shred cooled chicken (and cut pork into bite-sized pieces, if used); return to pot and warm through. Serves 14.

Exchanges: 1 bread, 2 meats, 1 vegetable

Tip: You can substitute half of the chicken with boneless pork chops for a tasty twist! (This does *not* alter the exchanges.)

CHICKEN AND DUMPLINGS

Contributed by Julia Faulk, Louisville, Mississippi

Boil chicken breasts in water until tender; remove from pot and reserve broth. Remove skin and bones from chicken; cut meat into pieces and return to broth. Bring chicken and broth to boil. Place flour in large bowl; create well in center. Crack egg into flour well; mix with small amount of flour. Add 1 cup chicken broth and mix well; place dough on floured cloth or board. Use rolling pin to roll dough until thin (about ⅛ inch thick). Cut dough into thin strips; pinch off in small pieces and drop into boiling broth, stirring as each piece is dropped in. If necessary, add more water (or fat-free chicken broth). Reduce heat to simmer; add butter and milk. Cover and cook 45 minutes, stirring once or twice. Serves 8.
Exchanges: 2 meats, 1 bread, 1 fat

4   large chicken breasts
Water, enough to cover chicken while boiling
2   c. flour
1   egg
½   stick light butter
1   c. nonfat milk
Salt and pepper to taste

CHICKEN AND PASTA

Contributed by Martha Rogers, Houston, Texas

Use nonstick skillet to brown chicken strips, onion and garlic in oil. Add tomato sauce, tomatoes, basil, oregano and thyme; bring to boil and then lower heat and simmer 30 minutes. Cook spaghetti as directed on package, omitting salt and fat; drain well. Pour sauce over spaghetti just prior to serving. Serves 4.
Exchanges: 4 meats, 1 bread, 1 ½ vegetables, ¾ fat

Tip: You can also make this dish with rice instead of spaghetti. Use ⅓ cup cooked rice per serving

1   lb. boneless, skinless chicken breasts, cut into strips
1   4-oz. pkg. spaghetti
¼   c. chopped onion
1   garlic clove, minced
1   tbsp. oil
1   8-oz. can tomato sauce
1   15-oz. can chopped tomatoes
1   tsp. basil
1   tsp. oregano
1   tsp. thyme

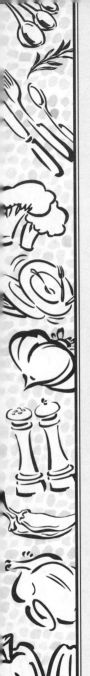

8 oz. boneless, skinless chicken
breasts, diced

3 c. cooked rice

1 large onion, chopped

½ c. chopped celery

¼ c. water or chicken bouillion

1 10.7-oz. can reduced-fat cream of
chicken soup

8 oz. Velveeta Light processed cheese
Salt and pepper to taste
Nonstick cooking spray

2 boneless skinless chicken breasts,
trimmed of all fat

2 c. water

2 stalks celery, diced

1 medium-sized sweet onion, chopped

2 carrots, sliced

½ c. brown rice

1 10.7-oz. can low-fat cream of
chicken soup

1 can low-fat crescent rolls (8 count)

CHICKEN AND RICE

Contributed by Judy Marshall, Gilmer, Texas

Note: *This dish freezes well, both before and after baking!*

Preheat oven to 350° F. Use medium nonstick skillet to sauté onion and celery in water or chicken bouillon. Add soup and cheese; stir until melted. Stir in rice and chicken; pour into 9x13-inch baking dish coated with cooking spray. Bake 30 minutes. Freezes well before or after baking. Serves 8.

Exchanges: 2 meats, 1 ½ breads, ½ vegetable, ½ fat

Tip: For variety, add 1 4½-ounce can diced green chiles and 1 8-ounce can water chestnuts (chopped). (This does *not* alter the exchanges.)

CHICKEN AND RICE POTPIE

Contributed by Carolyn Owen, Charlotte Court House, Virginia

Boil chicken until tender; remove meat to small bowl, reserving broth. Set meat aside to cool; pour broth into separate container and place both chicken and broth in refrigerator for 30 minutes or until fat surfaces to top of broth.

Preheat oven to 375° F. Remove chicken and broth from refrigerator; skim fat from broth. Return broth to pan and heat to boiling. Add celery and onion; simmer 10 minutes. Add carrots and cook 8 minutes more. Add chicken and rice; bring to a boil and let simmer 40 minutes or until rice is tender. Stir in cream of chicken soup and heat thoroughly; pour into 9x13-inch baking dish. Top with crescent rolls and bake until rolls are brown. Serves 8.

Exchanges: 2 meats, 2 breads, 1 fat

CHICKEN CASSEROLE

Contributed by Julie Anderson, Holland, Michigan

Cook noodles according to package directions, omitting salt and fat; drain and set aside. Preheat oven to 350° F. Combine cottage cheese, Parmesan cheese, ketchup and soy sauce in small bowl; blend well and set aside. In large bowl, combine noodles, chicken and cheese mixture; pour into 7x11-inch baking dish coated with cooking spray. Top with bread crumbs; bake uncovered 25 to 30 minutes. Serves 6.
Exchanges: 2 meats, 1 bread

1   6-oz. pkg. egg noodles
    (try no-yolk types)
9   oz. boneless, skinless chicken
    breasts, cooked and diced
½   c. low-fat cottage cheese
4   tbsp. Parmesan cheese
⅓   c. ketchup
1   tsp. soy sauce
¼   c. whole-wheat bread crumbs
    Nonstick cooking spray

CHICKEN CURRY

Contributed by Sheri Jackson, Okmulgee, Oklahoma

In large skillet, sauté chicken and onion in oil until chicken is browned. Stir in tomatoes and seasonings. Bring to boil; reduce heat and simmer covered 30 minutes. Serve over rice. Serves 8.
Exchanges: 3 meats, 2½ breads, 1 vegetable, ½ fat

1 ½ lbs. boneless, skinless chicken breasts
¼   c. chopped onion
2   tbsp. canola oil
1   28-oz. can garlic-and-onion
    seasoned tomatoes
1   tbsp. curry powder
½   tsp. salt
½   tsp. pepper
½   tsp. garlic powder
½   tsp. cayenne
½   tsp. paprika
½   tsp. chili powder
½   tsp. turmeric
½   tsp. ginger
⅛   tsp. ground cloves, to taste
6   c. cooked rice, warm

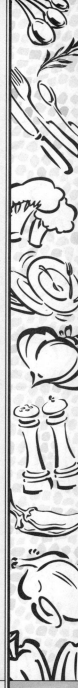

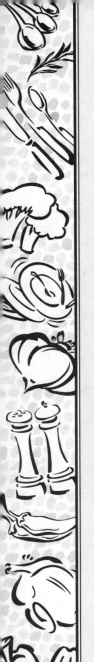

1 large whole chicken, thoroughly
washed and dried
⅓ c. chopped onion
⅓ c. chopped bell pepper
⅓ c. chopped celery
1 tsp. salt
¼ tsp. black pepper
Butter-flavored nonstick
cooking spray

2 boneless, skinless chicken breasts
2 tbsp. Italian-seasoned bread crumbs
1 tbsp. shredded Parmesan cheese
½ tsp. dried oregano
1 tbsp. lemon juice
1 small garlic clove, minced
Nonstick cooking spray

2 cooked boneless, skinless chicken
breasts, cut into bite-sized pieces
1 lb. bowtie or fusilli pasta
1 c. sun-dried tomatoes, julienne
3 tbsp. olive oil
1 c. Parmesan cheese

CHICKEN IN FOIL

Contributed by Judy Marshall, Gilmer, Texas

Preheat oven to 400° F. In small bowl, combine onion, bell pepper, celery, salt and pepper; mix well. Carefully stuff mixture into chicken cavity; coat outside of chicken with cooking spray and cover liberally with additional salt and pepper. Wrap tightly in heavy-duty foil; place in baking dish. Bake 1 ½ hours; open foil and bake 10 minutes more to brown skin. Peel off skin and discard prior to serving. Serves 6.

Exchanges: 2½ meats, ½ vegetable

CHICKEN PARMESAN ITALIANO

Contributed by Stephanie Cheves, Houston, Texas

Preheat oven to 425° F. Line baking sheet with foil; coat foil with cooking spray and set aside. In shallow dish, combine bread crumbs, cheese and oregano; mix well and set aside. In small bowl, combine lemon juice and garlic. Dredge chicken in juice mixture; coat with bread-crumb mixture and place on baking sheet. Lightly coat chicken with cooking spray; bake 15 to 20 minutes or until chicken is fork-tender and juice from chicken runs clear. Serves 2.

Exchanges: 4 meats, ½ bread, ½ fat

CHICKEN PASTA TOSS

Contributed by Barbara Bartlett, Kensington, Maryland

Cook pasta according to package directions, omitting salt and fat; drain and transfer to serving bowl. Toss with remaining ingredients; serve immediately. Serves 8.

Exchanges: 2 meat, 3 breads, 1 vegetable, 1 fat

CHICKEN REUBEN BAKE

Contributed by Mary Russell, Basin, Wyoming

6 boneless, skinless chicken breasts
1 14.5-oz. can sauerkraut, drained
6 oz. low-fat Swiss cheese
8 oz. fat-free Thousand Island salad dressing

> **Note:** *You can serve this with 2 slices light rye bread. (Add 1 bread exchange.)*

Preheat oven to 350° F. Cut each chicken breast in half lengthwise; place in 9x13-inch baking dish. Cover chicken with sauerkraut; layer slice of Swiss cheese over each breast. Spread dressing evenly over top. Bake 40 minutes covered with foil. Serves 12.

Exchanges: 4 ½ meats, ½ vegetable, ½ fat

CHICKEN SALAD

Contributed by Martha Rogers, Houston, Texas

2 c. cooked chicken
1 c. grapes, halved
½ c. finely chopped celery
¼ c. chopped nuts
¼ c. low-fat mayonnaise or Miracle Whip Light
90 low-fat saltine crackers

In a large bowl, combine chicken, grapes, celery, nuts and mayonnaise or Miracle Whip. Spread on crackers. Serves 15.

Exchanges: 1 meat, 1 bread, ½ fat

CHICKEN SPAGHETTI

Contributed by Anita Clayton, Lenoir City, Tennessee

3 skinless chicken-breast halves, bone in
1 12-oz. box spaghetti
3 stalks celery, chopped
1 large onion, chopped
1 large bell pepper, chopped
4 oz. sliced mushrooms
1 28-oz. can diced tomatoes
1 15-oz. can tomato sauce
1 tbsp. brown-sugar substitute
1 tsp. dried oregano
1 tsp. garlic salt

Cover chicken breasts in large pot with water; bring to boil and cook through. Remove chicken from pot; reserve broth. Allow chicken to cool to touch; once cooled, debone and chop into bite-sized pieces. In large nonstick skillet, sauté celery, onion and pepper until tender-crisp. Add mushrooms, tomatoes, tomato sauce, brown-sugar substitute, oregano, garlic salt and chicken pieces; simmer 30 to 45 minutes or until thickened.

While chicken is simmering, cook spaghetti using reserved broth, boiling until tender. Drain and serve with sauce. Serves 6.

Exchanges: 2 meats, 3 breads, 2 ½ vegetables

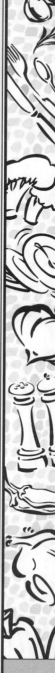

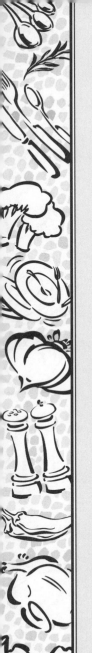

6   3-oz. boneless, skinless chicken
    breasts
3   egg whites
1   c. bread crumbs
1   c. grated Parmesan cheese
1   tsp. salt
1/4 tsp. black pepper
2   tbsp. parsley, minced
1   garlic clove, minced
1/4 oz. slivered almonds

2   boneless, skinless chicken breasts
12 manicotti pasta shells, cooked and
    cooled
1   c. fat-free sour cream
1   10.7-oz. can low-fat cream of
    chicken soup
1   10.7-oz. can low-fat cream of
    celery soup
1/4 c. Italian-seasoned bread crumbs
    Nonstick cooking spray

CHICKEN SUPREME
Contributed by Johnny Lewis, San Leon, Texas

Preheat oven to 350° F. Slightly beat egg whites in small bowl; set aside. Combine bread crumbs, cheese, salt, pepper, parsley, garlic and almonds (reserve a few for garnish) in shallow dish. Dip chicken breasts in egg whites; roll in bread-crumb mixture and arrange in 9x13-inch baking dish. Garnish with a few almond slivers. Bake 30 minutes. Serves 6.

Exchanges: 3 meats, 1/2 bread

CHICKEN-STUFFED MANICOTTI
Contributed by Patti McCoy, Fort Lupton, Colorado

Preheat oven to 350° F. Place chicken in microwave-safe bowl; microwave on high 8 to 10 minutes or until cooked through. Allow to cool; cut into bite-sized pieces. Combine chicken, sour cream, soups and bread crumbs in large bowl; stir well and spoon into manicotti. Arrange filled shells in 7x11-inch baking dish coated with cooking spray; spoon remaining mixture over top. Bake covered 25 minutes. Serves 6.

Exchanges: 1 1/2 meats, 2 breads

CHILI-CHICKEN NACHOS

Contributed by Connie Armstrong, Hattiesburg, Mississippi

In large bowl, combine chili powder, cumin, garlic powder, red pepper and oregano; add chicken strips and toss until strips are well coated. Sauté chicken strips in skillet coated with cooking spray using medium heat 7 to 8 minutes or until done. Add tomatoes; simmer 2 to 3 minutes and stir in cheese until melted. Spoon mixture evenly onto 4 plates, each with 1 ounce tortilla chips, 1 cup lettuce, 1 tablespoon sour cream and ¼ cup chopped green onions. Serves 4.
Exchanges: 2½ meats, 1½ breads, 1½ vegetables, ½ fat

8　oz. boneless, skinless chicken
　　breasts, cut into thin strips
2　tsp. chili powder
2　tsp. ground cumin
1　tsp. garlic powder
1　tsp. crushed red pepper
1½　tsp. fresh oregano
2　10-oz. can tomatoes with green
　　chiles, chunky style
½　c. low-fat cheddar cheese, shredded
4　oz. baked tortilla chips
4　c. shredded lettuce
4　tbsp. fat-free sour cream
1　c. chopped green onions
　　Nonstick cooking spray

CROCK-POT CHICKEN

Contributed by Blanche Gray, Huntsville, Alabama

Place frozen chicken breasts in bottom of Crock-Pot coated with cooking spray. Set Crock-Pot to low heat. In small bowl, combine sour cream, soup and soup mix; mix well and spread over chicken. Cook covered 6 to 7 hours. Serves 4.
Exchanges: 4 meats, ½ bread, ½ fat

4　skinless chicken-breast halves, frozen
1　16-oz. pkg. light sour cream
1　10.7-oz. can low-fat cream of
　　mushroom soup
1　envelope onion soup mix
　　Butter-flavored nonstick
　　cooking spray

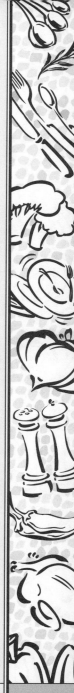

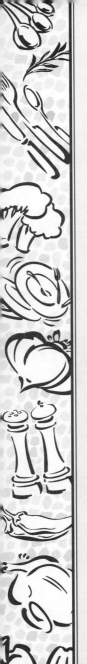

4 4-oz. boneless, skinless chicken
breasts
Salt and pepper to taste
1 c. low-fat sour cream
1 c. Italian-seasoned bread crumbs
Nonstick cooking spray

10 oz. boneless, skinless chicken
breasts, cooked and diced
9 oz. baked corn chips, broken
1 large onion, chopped
½ tsp. minced garlic
¾ c. chicken broth, divided
1 10.7-oz. can reduced-fat cream of
chicken soup
1 4.5-oz. can chopped green chiles
1 c. fat-free sour cream
¼ tsp. cumin
⅛ tsp. chili powder
1 c. grated cheddar cheese
1 bunch fresh cilantro, chopped
Nonstick cooking spray

CYNDI'S WATERFORD-LAKES CHICKEN

Contributed by Cyndi Crosby, Charlotte, North Carolina

Preheat oven to 375° F. Fillet breasts by running finger through tenderloin to flatten. Use mallet to flatten even more; salt and pepper to taste. Place sour cream and bread crumbs in separate shallow dishes. Dredge breasts through sour cream; roll in bread crumbs to coat and arrange on cooking sheet coated with cooking spray. Bake 15 to 20 minutes or until done. Serves 4.
Exchanges: 4 meats, 2 breads, 1 fat

DOUBLE T MEXICAN CHICKEN

Contributed by Judy Marshall, Gilmer, Texas

Preheat oven 350° F. Place broken chips in bottom of 9x13-inch dish coated with cooking spray; layer with chicken and set aside. In medium skillet, sauté onion and garlic in ¼ cup of broth until onion is transparent. Stir in soup, chiles, sour cream, cumin and chili powder; add remaining broth. Pour sauce over chicken; top with cheese and chopped cilantro. Bake uncovered 20 to 25 minutes. Serves 8.
Exchanges: 2 meats, 1½ breads, ½ fat

EASY CHICKEN FAJITA WRAPS

Contributed by Adina Collins, New Orleans, Louisiana

Rub chicken-breast pieces with seasoned salt and garlic powder; let sit 30 minutes. In small skillet, brown chicken, onion and bell pepper until chicken is cooked through and vegetables are tender-crisp. Arrange chicken mixture onto tortilla; add lettuce, tomato and salad dressing. Fold burrito style and cut in half. Serves 2.
Exchanges: ½ meat, ½ bread, ½ vegetable

1 oz. boneless, skinless chicken breast, cubed
  Seasoned salt to taste
¼ tsp. garlic powder
1 6-in. whole-wheat tortilla
¼ c. sliced onion
¼ c. sliced green bell pepper
¼ c. shredded lettuce
¼ c. sliced tomato
1 tbsp. low-fat ranch salad dressing

EASY CHICKEN SPAGHETTI

Contributed by Irene Sisk, Coal Hill, Arkansas

Prepare spaghetti according to package directions, omitting salt and fat; drain and set aside. Combine tomatoes with soups in saucepan; stir over medium heat until well blended and hot. Stir in cheese until melted; remove from heat and set aside. Combine chicken cubes with cooked pasta in 2-quart casserole dish; pour soup mixture over pasta, stirring to combine. Cover and heat in microwave 10 minutes or until sauce is bubbly. (You may use oven preheated to 350° F instead. Bake 30 minutes.) Serve immediately. Serves 6.
Exchanges: 2 meats, 2½ breads, 1 fat

12 oz. boneless, skinless chicken breasts, boiled and cubed
8 oz. spaghetti
1 10-oz. can diced tomatoes with green chiles
1 10.7-oz. can low-fat cream of chicken soup
1 10.7-oz. can low-fat cream of mushroom soup
8 oz. Velveeta Light processed cheese, cubed

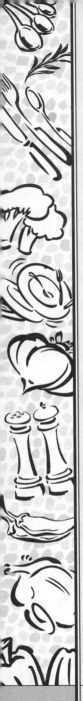

24 oz. boneless, skinless chicken thighs,
    cut into strips
1   c. flour
2   tbsp. paprika
1   tbsp. poultry seasoning
1   tbsp. onion powder
2   tbsp. salt
½   c. nonfat milk
    Nonstick cooking spray

1   lb. boneless, skinless chicken breasts
½   c. flour
2   tbsp. olive oil
6   garlic cloves, minced (or 2 heaping
    tsp. garlic powder)
1   c. chicken broth
⅓   c. balsamic vinegar
    Black pepper to taste

EASY OVEN-BAKED CHICKEN
Contributed by Carol Moore, Meridian, Mississippi

Preheat oven to 400° F. Cover large baking sheet with foil and coat heavily with cooking spray; set aside. Combine flour, paprika, poultry seasoning, onion powder and salt in shallow dish; stir well and set aside. Place chicken pieces in medium bowl; add milk and stir to coat. One at a time, dredge pieces through flour mixture to coat; shake off excess and place on baking sheet. Bake pieces 25 minutes; turn and bake 15 minutes more. (Note: If white flour is apparent when chicken is turned after first 25 minutes, spray with cooking spray before turning and cooking last 15 minutes.) Serves 8.
Exchanges: 1 meat, ½ bread

GARLIC CHICKEN FILLETS IN BALSAMIC VINEGAR
Contributed by Ann Hornbeak, Houston, Texas

Place flour in shallow dish; set aside. Preheat skillet and oil to medium-high heat. Dredge chicken breasts through flour; add to skillet and cook 2 to 3 minutes. Add garlic; turn chicken and cook 2 to 3 minutes more. Add broth, vinegar and pepper. Reduce heat to medium low; cover and cook 5 to 10 minutes more or until tender. Serves 6.
Exchanges: 2 meats, ½ bread, 1 fat

Tip: You can serve this scrumptious chicken over ½ cup rice or noodles per serving. (Add 1 bread exchange.)

GILMER'S BEST CHICKEN POTPIE

Contributed by Judy Marshall, Gilmer, Texas

Preheat oven to 350° F. Place one piecrust into deep-dish pie pan. Bake 7 to 9 minutes; remove from oven and set aside. In large bowl, combine vegetables with chicken, soup, garlic salt and pepper; mix well and pour into bottom cooked crust. Top with remaining crust; moisten fingers and press edges of crusts together to seal. Use knife to cut slits in top to vent; coat with cooking spray and sprinkle liberally with more garlic salt. Bake on foil-lined baking sheet 45 minutes; allow to cool 10 minutes before cutting. Serves 8.

Exchanges: 1 ½ meats, 1 bread, 1 ½ vegetables, 2 fats

- 3   boneless, skinless chicken breast halves, boiled and diced
- 2   deep-dish piecrusts, frozen
- 4   8-oz. cans mixed vegetables, drained and rinsed
- 1   10.7-oz. can low-fat cream of chicken soup
- 1   tsp. garlic salt
- 1   tsp. black pepper
      Butter-flavored nonstick cooking spray

GILMONT CHICKEN WITH ALFREDO SAUCE

Contributed by Judy Marshall, Gilmer, Texas

In a sauté pan, simmer onion, broccoli, carrots and mushrooms in chicken broth until just tender. Melt Parmesan cheese, cream cheese, margarine and milk in medium saucepan over medium heat, stirring occasionally to keep from scorching. Add garlic and chicken; salt and pepper to taste. Add more milk if necessary to thin; pour over fettucine. Serves 8.

Exchanges: 2 ½ meats, 1 bread, ½ vegetable, ½ milk, ½ fat

- 10 oz. boneless, skinless chicken breasts, boiled and diced
- 8   oz. fettuccine, cooked and warm
- 1   onion, chopped
- ½   head broccoli flowerets
- ½   c. julienne or grated carrots
- ½   lb. mushrooms, sliced or chopped
- ¼   c. chicken broth
- 1   c. freshly grated Parmesan cheese
- 1   8-oz. container fat-free cream cheese
- ¼   c. Brummel and Brown yogurt-based margarine
- 1   12-oz. can evaporated nonfat milk
- ¼   tsp. freshly ground garlic
      Salt and pepper to taste

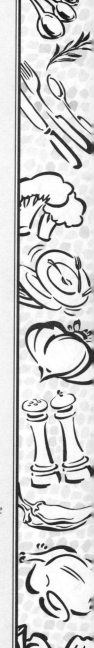

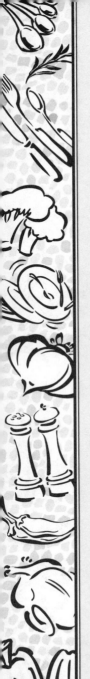

10 oz. boneless, skinless chicken
    breasts, cooked and diced
12 6-in. corn tortillas, torn into pieces
2 10.7-oz. cans reduced-fat cream of
    chicken soup
1 10-oz. can Rotel tomatoes
8 oz. Velveeta Light processed cheese
1 bell pepper, chopped
1 onion, chopped
¼ c. water or chicken broth
    Nonstick cooking spray

12 boneless, skinless chicken breasts
1½ tsp. salt, divided
4 c. bran flakes
24 low-fat saltine crackers
⅔ c. oats
1 c. flour
2 tbsp. Butter Buds (or other fat- and
    cholesterol-free butter-flavored
    granules)
1 tsp. garlic powder
    Butter-flavored nonstick cooking
    spray

MEXICAN CHICKEN

Contributed by Judy Marshall, Gilmer, Texas

Preheat oven to 350° F. In medium saucepan, heat soup, tomatoes and cheese until cheese is melted. Sauté bell pepper and onion in nonstick skillet with ¼ cup water or broth until tender. Stir into soup mixture; add chicken and tortillas. Pour into 9x13-inch baking dish coated with cooking spray. Bake 30 minutes. Serves 8.
Exchanges: 2 meats, 1½ breads, ½ vegetable

OVEN-FRIED CHICKEN

Contributed by Martha Norsworthy, Murray, Kentucky

Preheat oven to 350° F. Sprinkle ½ teaspoon salt over chicken breasts; set aside. Use rolling pin to crush bran flakes; set aside and crush crackers in same manner (important to crush flakes and crackers separately). In medium bowl, mix together crushed bran flakes, crushed crackers, remaining salt, oats, flour, Butter Buds and garlic powder. Pour about 1 cup mixture into shallow dish; set aside. Use paper towels to pat chicken breasts dry. Lightly coat 1 side of each breast with cooking spray and press into flake mixture; repeat with other side. Repeat until all breasts have been thoroughly coated twice, adding more mixture as needed. Arrange breasts on baking sheet coated with cooking spray; bake 15 minutes. Turn breasts and coat tops with cooking spray; return to oven. Cook 15 minutes more; turn over and coat again. Bake 45 minutes more. Serves 12.
Exchanges: 3 meats, 1 bread

Tip: This recipe makes approximately 3½ cups breading mixture but uses only about 2 cups. Place unused coating mix in an airtight container for future use.

RANCH-STYLE BREADED CHICKEN
Contributed by Peggy Grooms, Sherman, Texas

Preheat oven to 350° F. Place cheese, ranch dressing mix and cracker crumbs each in its own shallow dish or plate; set aside. Slightly beat egg whites in small bowl. One at a time, dip chicken breasts in egg whites; then roll in cheese, dressing mix and cracker crumbs. Place coated chicken breast on baking sheet coated with cooking spray; repeat with remaining breasts. Bake 35 to 40 minutes. Serves 4.
Exchanges: 4 meats, 1 bread

4 boneless, skinless chicken breasts
4 oz. fat-free cheddar cheese, shredded
1 1-oz. pkg. ranch dressing mix
20 fat-free saltine crackers, crushed
2 egg whites
Nonstick cooking spray

SANDY'S CHICKEN POTPIE
Contributed by Sandy Bundick, Hitchcock, Texas

Preheat oven to 350° F. Brown chicken in skillet coated with cooking spray; cut into bite-sized pieces. Add chicken broth, vegetables, soup, corn and herb seasoning; heat through and add salt and pepper to taste. Pour into piecrust; bake 40 to 45 minutes or until edge of crust is browned. Serves 6.
Exchanges: 2 meats, 1 bread, ½ vegetable, 1½ fats

9 oz. boneless, skinless chicken breasts
⅔ c. fat-free chicken broth
1 29-oz. can mixed vegetables
1 10 ¾-oz. can fat-free cream of chicken soup
1 c. white corn kernels
¼ tsp. chicken herb seasoning
Salt and pepper to taste
1 frozen piecrust, thawed
Nonstick cooking spray

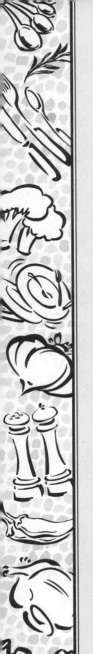

2 lbs. boneless, skinless chicken breasts
½ c. (2 oz.) sesame seeds
½ c. fine bread crumbs
¼ tsp. garlic powder
2 tsp. paprika
1 tsp. salt
¼ tsp. pepper
1 egg, beaten
½ c. nonfat milk
    Nonstick cooking spray

8 boneless, skinless chicken-breast
    halves, diced
3 4.5-oz. cans chopped green chiles
1 15.5-oz. can pinto beans, rinsed
    and drained
1 14.5-oz. can diced tomatoes
1 11-oz. can corn, drained
1 14.5-oz. can tomatoes with
    green chiles
1 10.7-oz. can low-fat cream of
    chicken soup
1 large onion, chopped
1 tsp. chicken bouillon
1 tsp. minced garlic
¼ tsp. cumin
¼ tsp. oregano
¾ c. fat-free sour cream
¾ c. grated cheddar cheese
24 baked tortilla chips
    Chopped green onion to taste
    Chopped fresh cilantro to taste

SESAME BAKED CHICKEN

Contributed by Ann Hornbeak, Houston, Texas

Preheat over to 325° F. In shallow dish, combine sesame seeds, bread crumbs, garlic powder, paprika, salt and pepper; set aside. In large bowl, whisk together egg and milk. Dredge chicken in egg mixture; coat with sesame seed mixture and arrange pieces on baking sheet coated with cooking spray. Bake 1 hour and 15 minutes or until crisp. Serves 8.
Exchanges: 4 meats, ½ bread, 1 fat

SLOW "SOUPER" CHILE-CHICKEN

Contributed by Judy Marshall, Gilmer, Texas

Place chicken, chiles, pinto beans, diced tomatoes, corn, tomatoes with chiles, chicken soup, onion, bouillion, garlic, cumin and oregano in order into slow cooker set to low heat. Cover and cook 7 to 8 hours (or 4 hours on high setting). Serve each topped with 1 tablespoon sour cream, 1 tablespoon cheese, 2 broken tortilla chips, and chopped green onion and cilantro to taste. Serves 12.
Exchanges: 2 meats, ½ bread, 1 vegetable

SLOW-COOKED ORANGE CHICKEN

Contributed by Martha Rogers, Houston, Texas

Combine chicken, orange juice, celery, bell pepper, onion, salt and pepper in slow cooker; cook on low setting 4 hours or until meat juices run clear.

Combine cornstarch and water until smooth; stir into slow cooker; cover and change setting to high. Cook 30 to 40 minutes. Serve each over ⅓ cup rice. Serves 4.

Exchanges: 3 meats, 1 bread, ½ vegetable, 1½ fruits

4   3-oz. boneless, skinless chicken breasts
3   c. orange juice
1   c. chopped celery
1   c. chopped green bell pepper
¼   c. chopped onion
½   tsp. salt
¼   tsp. black pepper
3   tbsp. cornstarch
3   tbsp. cold water
1⅓ c. cooked rice

SMOTHERED ITALIAN CHICKEN

Contributed by Peggy Grooms, Sherman, Texas

Pour ½ cup salad dressing in shallow dish. Place chicken in dish, turning to coat both sides. Cover and refrigerate at least 4 hours.

Preheat oven to 350° F. Cook marinated chicken in large preheated nonstick skillet coated with cooking spray until golden brown on each side. Arrange pieces in 7x11-inch baking dish coated with cooking spray; layer with onion slices and top with remaining dressing and water. Bake 30 to 35 minutes. Serves 4.

Exchanges: 4 meats, ½ vegetable

4   4-oz. boneless, skinless chicken breasts
¾   c. low-fat Italian salad dressing, divided
1   large onion, sliced
¼   c. water
    Nonstick cooking spray

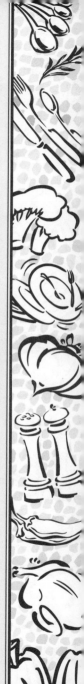

16 oz. boneless, skinless chicken
 breasts, flattened with mallet
3 ½ oz. roasted red peppers
 2 oz. chopped olives
 1 garlic clove, minced
 2 tbsp. minced onion
 1 tsp. basil
 4 tsp. olive oil
1 ¼ c. dry white wine
 (or water, if desired)

 1 lb. boneless, skinless chicken breasts,
 cut into 1-in. pieces
 1 tbsp. cooking sherry
 4 tbsp. low-sodium soy sauce, divided
 Egg substitute to equal 1 egg
 ¼ tsp. black pepper
 ¼ tsp. garlic powder
 ¼ c. plus 2 tbsp. cornstarch
 2 tbsp. olive oil
 1 15-oz. can pineapple chunks in juice
 Water
 ½ c. sugar substitute
 ¼ c. ketchup
 ¼ c. vinegar
 1 medium bell pepper, cut into 1-in.
 pieces

STUFFED CHICKEN BREASTS

Contributed by Stephanie Cheves, Houston, Texas

Cut peppers into pieces large enough to cover center of each chicken breast; top each breast with 1 pepper and set aside. Combine olives, garlic, onion and basil on cutting board; chop together very fine and spoon over pepper-topped chicken. Fold chicken over stuffing; secure with toothpick. Heat oil in large skillet over low heat. Layer rolled chicken breasts across skillet; increase heat to medium and cook on each side until browned. (Keep stirring so breasts don't stick.) Add wine (or water); bring to boil and reduce heat. Cover and simmer 10 to 15 minutes or until chicken is tender and cooked through. Serve with pan juices. Serves 4.
Exchanges: 4 meats, ½ vegetable, 1 fat

SWEET-AND-SOUR CHICKEN

Contributed by Ouida Donald, Louisville, Mississippi

In large bowl, combine cooking sherry, 3 tablespoons soy sauce, egg substitute, pepper, garlic powder and ¼ cup cornstarch; mix well. Add chicken; stir to coat. Preheat oil in electric skillet set to 375° F. Stir-fry chicken until lightly browned and set aside. Drain juice from pineapple into measuring cup and add enough water to bring amount to 1 cup. Add 2 tablespoons cornstarch; stir well. Combine pineapple-juice mixture, sugar substitute, ketchup, vinegar and 1 tablespoon soy sauce in medium saucepan; bring mixture to a boil and stir in bell pepper and chicken. Cook until thoroughly heated. Serves 6.
Exchanges: 3 meats, 1 bread, 1 fat

Tip: You can serve this with ⅓ cup cooked rice per serving. (Add 1 bread exchange.)

TACO CHICKEN CASSEROLE

Contributed by Kelly Fisher, Houston, Texas

4   3-oz. boneless, skinless chicken
    breasts
1   envelope taco seasoning mix
1   15-oz. can Rotel tomatoes
1   8-oz. can sliced black olives
4   tbsp. fat-free sour cream or plain
    yogurt

Preheat oven to 350° F. Coat chicken breasts with taco seasoning and place in baking dish. Top with Rotel tomatoes (with liquid from can) and black olives. Cover and bake 25 minutes or until chicken is no longer pink in the middle. Serve topped with sour cream or yogurt. Serves 4.
Exchanges: 4 meats, ½ bread, ½ vegetable, ½ fat

TURKEY BARBECUE

Contributed by Dick Porter, Hartsville, South Carolina

1   10- to 12-lb. whole turkey, skin
    removed and cut up
1   tbsp. all-purpose flour
2   18-oz. bottles barbecue sauce

Preheat oven to 350° F. Place flour inside large oven-cooking bag; shake well. Place bag in large roasting pan at least 2 inches deep. Arrange turkey pieces in bag; add one bottle barbecue sauce. Close bag and seal. Use knife to create 6 half-inch slits in top of bag. Bake 2½ to 3 hours or until very tender; remove bag from oven. Remove turkey from bag; set aside to cool. Discard bag and drippings. When meat is cool to the touch, remove bones and discard. Chop meat into pieces; return to roasting pan and stir in remaining bottle of barbecue sauce. Cover and bake 20 to 25 minutes more or until thoroughly heated. Serves 13.
Exchanges: 4 meats

8 oz. lean turkey Italian sausage

2 small zucchini, quartered lengthwise

1 medium onion, chopped

2 garlic cloves, chopped

1 14½-oz. can stewed tomatoes

3 oz. uncooked spaghetti, broken into 1-in. pieces (about ¾ c. after breaking)

½ c. water

¼ c. grated Parmesan cheese

Nonstick cooking spray

TURKEY-SAUSAGE AND SPAGHETTI CASSEROLE

Contributed by Patricia Welker, Farmington, Illinois

Preheat oven to 375° F. In large nonstick skillet coated with cooking spray, cook sausage over medium heat, breaking up with a spoon. When meat is almost done, add zucchini and onion; continue cooking 10 minutes or until zucchini is tender-crisp. Drain and then rinse with hot water if desired. Add garlic to skillet; cook 1 minute more. Stir in tomatoes, spaghetti and water; transfer mixture to 11x7-inch baking dish coated with cooking spray. Cover with foil; bake 30 minutes. Sprinkle with Parmesan cheese and let stand 5 minutes before serving. Serves 6.

Exchanges: 1½ meats, ½ bread, ½ vegetable, 1 fat

SIDE DISHES

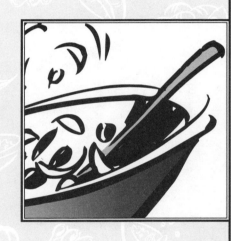

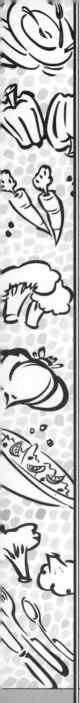

An Important Note

The terms "artificial sweetener" and "sugar substitute" do not refer to the same products in the following recipes!

Artificial sweeteners refer to sweeteners measured by the packet (e.g., Equal and Sweet'N Low). Sugar substitutes refer to sweeteners that can be measured as if measuring sugar for cooking or baking (e.g., Splenda).

2 large tomatoes, halved
2 tsp. oil
½ tsp. fresh parsley (or ¼ tsp. dried)
¼ tsp. oregano
¼ tsp. basil
   Nonstick cooking spray

Side Dishes

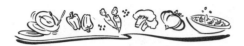

COOKED DISHES

BAKED TOMATOES
Contributed by Ann Hornbeak, Houston, Texas

Preheat oven to 350° F. Arrange tomato halves in small baking dish coated with cooking spray. Drizzle with oil; sprinkle with parsley, oregano and basil. Bake 20 to 30 minutes. Serves 4.

Exchanges: 1 vegetable, ½ fat

BLACK-EYED PEAS

Contributed by Frances Ventress, New Orleans, Louisiana

Place peas in large pot with water, broth, bay leaves and red-pepper flakes; cook 1 hour over low heat. Add onion, garlic, jalapeño pepper, cilantro, coriander, thyme, basil and oil; cook 1 to 1½ hours more or to desired consistency, adding water as needed to cover peas. Salt may be added to taste, if desired. Serves 6.

Exchanges: 2½ meats, 3 breads, ½ vegetable, 1 fat

1 lb. black-eyed peas, soaked overnight in water

6 c. water

2 14½-oz. cans low-fat, low-sodium chicken broth

3 large bay leaves
Pinch red-pepper flakes

1 large onion, chopped

1½ tbsp. minced garlic

½ large jalapeño pepper, seeded and chopped

¼ c. chopped fresh cilantro

½ tsp. ground coriander

½ tsp. chopped fresh thyme

1 pinch dried basil

2 tbsp. olive oil
Salt to taste (optional)

BLUE-RIBBON VEGETABLES

Contributed by Kay Smith, Roscoe, Texas

Preheat oven to 350° F. Use margarine to brown Rice Krispies in skillet over medium heat; set aside. Place vegetables in 9x13-inch baking dish; set aside. In medium bowl, combine cream of celery soup, sour cream, milk and onion soup mix; pour over vegetables. Gently press browned Rice Krispies over top; bake 30 minutes. Serves 8.

Exchanges: ½ bread, 1 vegetable, 1 fat

2 16-oz. pkgs. frozen broccoli, carrots and cauliflower, cooked and drained

3 c. Rice Krispies

3 tbsp. reduced-calorie margarine

1 10.7-oz. can cream of celery soup

1 8-oz. container light sour cream

8 oz. nonfat milk

1 envelope onion soup mix

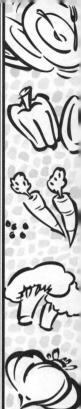

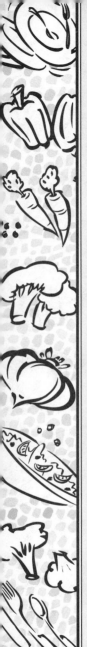

½ lb. lean ground beef
½ lb. ground pork
1 lb. ground turkey breast
1 large cabbage head
1 tbsp. salt or Mrs. Dash seasoning
½ tsp. black pepper
2 small onions, minced
1 garlic clove, minced
1 c. cooked brown rice
1 15-oz. can tomatoes
Butter-flavored nonstick
cooking spray

1½ c. cauliflower flowerets
¼ c. water
1 c. sliced carrots (⅛ in. thick)

1 15¼-oz. can corn, drained
1 15-oz. can creamed corn
1 16-oz. container light sour cream
2 eggs, beaten
1 8½-oz. package cornbread mix
2 tbsp. butter, melted
1 tsp. sugar
Dash salt
Nonstick cooking spray

CABBAGE ROLLS

Contributed by Evelyn Bailey, New Orleans, Louisiana

Preheat oven to 350° F. Gently remove 8 large leaves from cabbage and wash thoroughly. Place leaves in saucepan with enough boiling water to measure 1-inch thickness in pan. Cover and simmer 5 minutes; drain and lay out on flat surface. Combine meats in pan coated with cooking spray; sauté until browned. Remove from heat; add salt, pepper, onions, garlic and rice; mix well. Fill each cabbage leaf with an equal amount of mixture; roll up leaves, folding ends toward center and securing with toothpick. Place rolls in baking dish coated with cooking spray; pour tomatoes over top. Cover and bake 45 minutes. Remove toothpicks before serving. Serves 8.
Exchanges: 3½ meats, ½ bread, ½ vegetable, 1½ fats

CAULIFLOWER AND CARROTS

Contributed by Ann Hornbeak, Houston, Texas

Place cauliflower and water in microwave-safe dish; microwave on high 2 to 3 minutes. Add carrots; microwave 2 to 4½ minutes more. Serve warm. Serves 4.
Exchanges: 1 vegetable

CREAMY CORN CASSEROLE

Contributed by Ann Hornbeak, Houston, Texas

Preheat oven to 350° F. Combine corn, sour cream, eggs, cornbread mix, butter, sugar and salt in large bowl; mix well. Pour into 9x13-inch baking dish coated with cooking spray. Bake uncovered 1 hour. Let sit 10 minutes before serving. Serves 16.
Exchanges: 1 bread, 1 fat

CRISPY ZUCCHINI COINS

Contributed by Sheri Jackson, Okmulgee, Oklahoma

Preheat oven to 450° F. Combine bread crumbs, Parmesan cheese and pepper in large shallow dish; mix well and set aside. Dip zucchini slices in egg whites; dredge through bread-crumb mixture and arrange in single layer on baking sheet coated with cooking spray. Bake 20 minutes; turn over and bake 15 minutes more or until crispy and browned. Serves 4.

Exchanges: ½ meat, 1 bread, ¾ vegetable

3 c. thinly sliced zucchini
½ c. seasoned bread crumbs
3 tbsp. Parmesan cheese
¼ tsp. pepper
2 egg whites, lightly beaten
Nonstick cooking spray

HOT GARLIC-ROASTED POTATOES

Contributed by Frances Ventress, New Orleans, Louisiana

In baking pan coated with cooking spray, combine potatoes, oil and spices; toss to coat evenly. Cover pan with foil; use knife to make small puncture in middle to vent. Roast 30 minutes; remove foil and discard. Lightly stir and bake 15 minutes more or until tender. Serves 6.

Exchanges: 2 breads, 1 fat

6 5-oz. potatoes, peeled and quartered
2 tbsp. olive oil
2 tbsp. ground coriander
2 tbsp. chopped fresh cilantro
1 tbsp. minced garlic
Pinch dried basil
Nonstick cooking spray

ITALIAN VEGETARIAN CASSEROLE

Contributed by Kelly McQueen, Gilmer, Texas

Preheat oven to 350° F. Combine vegetables, garlic, tomatoes, seasoning and Parmesan cheese in large bowl; toss to thoroughly coat. Pour into 9x13-inch baking dish coated with cooking spray; sprinkle with mozzarella cheese, if desired. Bake 45 to 55 minutes. Serves 10.

Exchanges: 1 meat, 1 vegetable

8 c. mixed vegetables (your choice)
1 tbsp. minced garlic
2 14½-oz. cans diced tomatoes
1 tbsp. Chef Paul Prudhomme's Seafood Magic seasoning
½ c. grated Parmesan cheese
4 oz. grated mozzarella cheese (optional)
Nonstick cooking spray

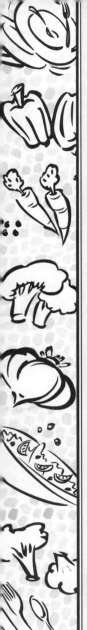

3 medium zucchini, sliced
1 tbsp. olive oil
½ medium white onion, chopped
2 to 3 garlic cloves, minced
1 pint cherry tomatoes, halved
1 11-oz. can corn
1 tsp. oregano
6 tsp. grated Parmesan cheese

1 lb. baby carrots
2 tbsp. reduced-calorie margarine
1 tbsp. lemon juice
½ tsp. garlic powder
½ tsp. dried basil
Dash pepper

2 c. nonfat cottage cheese
1 c. nonfat sour cream
¼ c. egg substitute
¾ tsp. salt
¼ tsp. garlic powder
Pepper to taste
2 c. grated, reduced-fat cheddar cheese
1⅔ c. macaroni, cooked and drained
Nonstick cooking spray

ITALIAN ZUCCHINI SAUTÉ
Contributed by Cheryl Milligan, Tracy, California

Preheat skillet and oil on medium-high heat. Sauté onion and garlic until tender-crisp. Add zucchini, tomatoes, corn and oregano; stir well. Cover and simmer 10 minutes on low heat or until zucchini is tender-crisp. Sprinkle with Parmesan cheese and serve hot. Serves 8.

Exchanges: ½ meat, ½ bread, 1 vegetable, ½ fat

LEMON AND BASIL CARROTS
Contributed by Alyce Amussen, Silver Spring, Maryland

Boil carrots in medium saucepan with salted water 20 minutes or until tender; drain and remove from pan. Set aside. In same pan, melt margarine; stir in lemon juice, garlic powder, basil and pepper. Add carrots, cover and toss until carrots are well coated. Let sit 3 minutes before serving. Serves 8.

Exchanges: 1 vegetable, ½ fat

MACARONI AND CHEESE
Contributed by Gretchen Brown, Forest Grove, Oregon

Preheat oven to 350° F. Combine cottage cheese, sour cream, egg substitute, salt, garlic powder and pepper in large bowl; stir in cheddar cheese and mix well. Add macaroni and stir until coated. Transfer to 2 ½ -quart casserole dish coated with cooking spray. Bake uncovered 25 to 30 minutes or until heated through. Garnish with paprika, if desired. Serves 8.

Exchanges: 2 meats, 1 bread

NOT-SO-SWEET POTATOES

Contributed by Pauline Hines, New Orleans, Louisiana

Preheat oven to 400° F. Place potatoes in 3- to 5-quart Dutch oven; bake 1 hour or until tender. Remove from oven and allow to cool.

Combine cinnamon, nutmeg, vanilla, maple syrup, dried fruit, sunflower seeds and almonds. Arrange cooked potatoes on serving dish, slit with knife and evenly distribute topping mixture over each. Serves 6.

Exchanges: 2½ breads, ½ fat

2	lb. sweet potatoes, washed
1 ½	tsp. ground cinnamon
1 ½	tsp. nutmeg
1 ½	tsp. vanilla extract
⅓	c. maple syrup
⅓	c. Sunmaid dried fruit medley
2	tbsp. sunflower seeds
2	tbsp. almonds

OKRA AND TOMATOES

Contributed by Adina Collins, New Orleans, Louisiana

In medium pot coated with cooking spray, sauté onion, bell pepper and garlic until soft. Add okra and stir well; let cook 20 minutes over low heat. Add tomatoes, seasoned salt, Italian seasoning and parsley; cook on medium 20 minutes more or until tender. Add shrimp and cook until shrimp are pink. Serves 4 to 6.

Exchanges: 1 meat, 1½ vegetables

1	lb. frozen okra, thawed
1	14 ½-oz. can crushed tomatoes
1	small onion, chopped
½	bell pepper, chopped
2	tbsp. garlic
	Seasoned salt to taste
	Italian seasoning to taste
	Parsley to taste
½	lb. shrimp, shelled and deveined
	Nonstick cooking spray

OKRA SUCCOTASH

Contributed by Judy Marshall, Gilmer, Texas

Rinse okra under running water; drain and combine with remaining ingredients in large skillet. Cover and simmer 15 to 20 minutes. Season to taste. Serves 6.

Exchanges: ½ bread, 1½ vegetables

3	c. sliced okra (fresh or frozen)
1	15.2-oz. can corn, drained
1	14 ½-oz. can diced tomatoes, any style
1	large onion, chopped

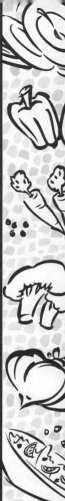

SIDE DISHES

Cooked Dishes

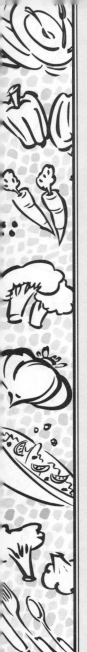

2 ½ c. sliced carrots
¼ c. water
½ c. unsweetened orange juice
1 tbsp. cornstarch
2 tbsp. margarine
1 medium orange, diced or sectioned

2 medium green tomatoes
  (or small zucchini or yellow squash)
2 ½ tbsp. flour
Salt and pepper to taste
Butter-flavored nonstick cooking
spray

3 medium potatoes, sliced
1 large onion, sliced
Salt and pepper to taste
Butter-flavored nonstick
cooking spray

SIDE DISHES

Cooked Dishes

ORANGE-GLAZED CARROTS

Contributed by Ann Hornbeak, Houston, Texas

Microwave carrots and water in microwave-safe dish on high 8 to 10 minutes; drain liquid into measuring cup. Add orange juice and enough water to make 1 cup of liquid. Remove carrots from pan; set aside. Pour orange juice mixture into same dish; stir in cornstarch and mix well. Microwave on high 1 ½ minutes; stir and microwave 1 ½ minutes more. Add carrots, margarine and orange pieces; mix well and microwave 2 minutes more. Serves 6.

Exchanges: 1 vegetable, ½ fruit, 1 fat

OVEN-FRIED GREEN TOMATOES OR SQUASH

Contributed by Ronda Robbs, Fredericktown, Missouri

Preheat oven to broil. Combine flour, salt and pepper in a quart-sized storage bag. Add several slices of tomato or squash to bag and shake to coat. Remove slices and place on baking sheet coated with cooking spray. Repeat until all slices are coated. Lightly spray slices with cooking spray; broil until brown. Turn over and spray again with cooking spray; broil until brown on second side. Serve immediately. Serves 2.

Exchanges: ½ bread, 1 vegetable

OVEN-FRIED POTATOES

Contributed by Georgia Senn, Gilmer, Texas

Preheat oven to 375° F. Place sliced potatoes and onion into baking pan generously coated with cooking spray. Salt and pepper to taste; coat with cooking spray. Bake 35 to 40 minutes, stirring occasionally. Serves 6.

Exchanges: 1 bread, ½ vegetable

PEAS AND ASPARAGUS

Contributed by Irene Bell, Aynor, South Carolina

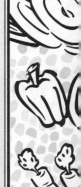

Add peas, asparagus, margarine, mint, garlic salt and pepper to boiling water in large saucepan. Bring to boil and reduce heat; cover and simmer 10 minutes or until asparagus is tender-crisp. Drain and serve immediately. Serves 6.
Exchanges: 1 bread, 1 vegetable, 1 fat

2   10-oz. pkgs. frozen peas
¾   lb. fresh asparagus, cut into 1-in. pieces
3   tbsp. reduced-fat margarine
1   tbsp. minced mint leaves
¾   tsp. garlic salt (optional)
    Dash pepper
½   c. water

PEPPERED SUGAR-SNAP PEAS

Contributed by Ann Hornbeak, Houston, Texas

Combine all ingredients in 1-quart casserole dish; cover and microwave on high 3 minutes. Stir and replace cover; microwave 3 minutes more. Let stand 2 minutes. Serves 4.
Exchanges: 1 vegetable, ½ fat

1   8-oz. pkg. frozen sugar-snap peas
1   small red bell pepper, sliced into thin strips
1   celery stalk, sliced thin diagonally
2   tsp. margarine

PINEAPPLE CARROTS

Contributed by Ann Hornbeak, Houston, Texas

Combine pineapple, water and salt in saucepan. Add carrots; cover and simmer 12 to 15 minutes or until tender. Reduce heat to low. In small bowl or cup, combine reserved pineapple juice and cornstarch, stirring with fork until smooth. Pour mixture slowly into saucepan, stirring constantly. Cook over low heat until bubbly, stirring constantly. Stir in parsley; season to taste with salt and pepper. Serves 4.
Exchanges: ½ vegetable, ½ fruit

1   8-oz. can crushed pineapple in juice, drained with 2 tbsp. juice reserved
4   large carrots, julienned
½   c. water
¼   tsp. salt
1   tsp. cornstarch
1   tbsp. snipped parsley
    Salt and pepper to taste

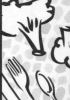

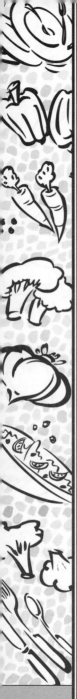

2 lbs. pinto beans, rinsed
10 qts. water
6 whole garlic cloves
1 large onion, coarsely chopped
1 tbsp. chili powder
1 tbsp. Creole seasoning
1 tbsp. goya adobo
1 tsp. salt

4 c. shredded potatoes
4 whole eggs
12 egg whites
Salt and pepper to taste
Nonstick cooking spray

PINTO BEANS Á LA JUAN

Contributed by Johnny Lewis, San Leon, Texas

Bring all ingredients to boil in 3-gallon pot. Boil gently 1 ½ hours; taste for seasoning; add more if desired. Continue boiling gently 3 ½ hours more. Serves 24.
Exchanges: 1 bread

Tip: For added flavor with a cilantro flare, add the following ingredients when beans are tender:
- 2 medium bell peppers, coarsely chopped;
- 4 firm tomatoes, coarsely chopped;
- 1 large yellow onion, coarsely chopped; and
- 1 cilantro bunch, rinsed and tied (discard when done cooking).

(Add ½ vegetable exchange.)

QUICK POTATO PANCAKES

Contributed by Robbie Kribell, Buena Park, California

Note: *For a tasty variation that won't alter the exchanges, add 1 cup chopped mushrooms!*

In medium bowl, combine potatoes, eggs and egg whites; mix well and pour into preheated skillet coated with cooking spray. Cook 5 minutes over medium-high heat, turning once halfway through cooking to brown both sides. Salt and pepper to taste. Serves 4.
Exchanges: 2 meats, 2 breads

Tip: Add 1 cup shredded or finely diced vegetable(s) of choice (e.g., bell pepper, carrots or onion) to add variety to this recipe. (Add ½ vegetable exchange.)

SPICY SWEET POTATOES

Contributed by Sheri Jackson, Okmulgee, Oklahoma

Preheat oven to 400° F. In large freezer bag (or bowl with lid), combine sweet potatoes and oil, tossing to coat potatoes. Add brown sugar, chili powder, salt and cayenne pepper; toss to coat. Arrange coated potatoes in 7x11-inch baking dish coated with cooking spray. Bake uncovered 40 to 45 minutes or until tender, stirring every 15 minutes. Serves 8.
Exchanges: 1 bread, ½ fat

3 large sweet potatoes, peeled and cubed
2 tbsp. olive oil
2 tbsp. brown sugar
1 tsp. chili powder
½ tsp. salt
¼ tsp. cayenne pepper
Nonstick cooking spray

SQUASH BAKE

Contributed by Judy Marshall, Gilmer, Texas

Preheat oven to 350° F. In medium saucepan, boil squash, onion and bell pepper in small amount of salted water until soft. Drain well; mash and drain again. Add chiles, salt, pepper, soup, water chestnuts and cheese to vegetables; stir to combine and season to taste. Pour into 9x13-inch baking dish coated with cooking spray. Bake 30 minutes. Serves 8.
Exchanges: 1 meat, 2 vegetables, ½ fat

3 ½ lbs. yellow squash, coarsely chopped
1 onion, chopped
1 bell pepper, chopped
1 4-oz. can green chiles, drained and chopped
Salt and pepper to taste
1 10.7-oz. can reduced-fat cream of chicken soup
1 8-oz. can water chestnuts, drained and chopped
8 oz. Velveeta Light processed cheese
Nonstick cooking spray

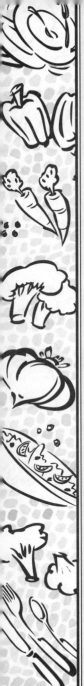

1 lb. fresh yellow squash, thinly sliced
1 medium bell pepper, chopped
2 fresh tomatoes, chopped
   (or 1 10-oz. can Rotel tomatoes,
   drained and diced)
4 oz. cheddar cheese, grated
   Salt and pepper to taste
1 10.7-oz. can reduced-fat cream of
   chicken soup
   Nonstick cooking spray

2 large sweet potatoes, peeled and sliced
2 large apples, sliced
½ c. finely chopped pecans
6 oz. frozen orange juice concentrate,
   thawed
¼ c. brown-sugar substitute
½ c. reduced-fat margarine

1 medium zucchini, sliced
¾ c. soft bread crumbs, divided
1 large onion, thinly sliced
2 medium tomatoes, peeled and sliced
½ tsp. salt
¼ tsp. pepper
¼ tsp. fresh oregano
   Butter-flavored nonstick
   cooking spray

SIDE DISHES

Cooked Dishes

SQUASH CASSEROLE
Contributed by Judy Marshall, Gilmer, Texas

Preheat oven to 350° F. Layer squash, bell pepper, tomatoes and cheese in 9x13-inch baking dish coated with cooking spray. Salt and pepper to taste; spread soup evenly over top. Cover with foil and bake 1 hour and 15 minutes. Serves 8.
Exchanges: ½ meat, 1 vegetable, 1 fat

Tip: This is great without the cheese if you'd like to omit the meat and fat exchanges!

SWEET POTATO AND APPLE CASSEROLE
Contributed by Lynda Martinaz, Madison, Mississippi

Preheat oven to 350° F. Place ½ of sweet potatoes in bottom of shallow 2-quart casserole dish. Add layer of ½ of apples; sprinkle ½ of pecans over top. Repeat layers; set aside. In small bowl, combine orange juice concentrate, brown-sugar substitute and margarine; mix well and pour into casserole dish. Cover and bake 45 to 60 minutes or until tender. Serves 8.
Exchanges: ½ bread, ½ fruit, 2 fats

ZUCCHINI CASSEROLE
Contributed by Irene Bell, Aynor, South Carolina

Preheat oven to 350° F. Place ½ cup bread crumbs in bottom of 1½-quart casserole dish coated with cooking spray. Layer ½ of zucchini, onion and tomatoes in order over bread crumbs; sprinkle with salt, pepper and oregano to taste. Repeat layers of veggies and seasonings. Top with remaining bread crumbs and generously coat with cooking spray. Bake uncovered 1 hour or until vegetables are tender. Serves 6.
Exchanges: ½ bread, 1 vegetable

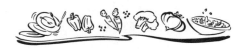

SALADS, SLAWS
AND MARINATED VEGGIES

BEET SALAD

Contributed by Carolyn Holmes, Zwolle, Louisiana

Combine beet and pineapple juices in measuring cup; add water if needed to equal 1½ cups liquid. Add juices, gelatin, sugar substitute and salt in saucepan and heat until gelatin is dissolved; remove from heat and stir in beets and pineapple. Pour into 9x9-inch baking dish. Refrigerate at least 1 hour.

In small bowl, combine mayonnaise, celery and onions; mix well. Spread on chilled salad just prior to serving to prevent red color from bleeding through. Serves 5.

Exchanges: 1 vegetable, ½ fruit, 1 fat

1   15-oz. can beets, drained (juice reserved)
1   8-oz. can crushed pineapple in juice, drained (juice reserved)
1   .3-oz. box sugar-free lemon-flavored gelatin
¼ c. sugar substitute
    Pinch salt
¾ c. low-fat mayonnaise
½ c. diced celery
5   green onions, finely chopped

BROCCOLI SALAD

Contributed by Janet Bayless, Clinton, Tennessee

Brown bacon in skillet; drain and set aside to cool. In large salad bowl, combine broccoli, onion, raisins, water chestnuts, Miracle Whip, vinegar and sweetener. Crumble bacon on top of salad and serve. Serves 6.

Exchanges: 1 vegetable, ⅓ fruit, ⅓ fat

4   slices turkey bacon (or 2 tbsp. imitation bacon bits)
4   c. coarsely chopped broccoli florets
½ c. chopped onion
¼ c. raisins
1   8-oz. can water chestnuts, drained
½ c. fat-free Miracle Whip
2   tbsp. vinegar
4   packets artificial sweetener

SIDE DISHES

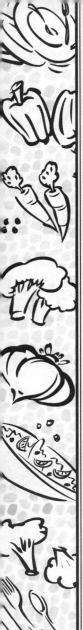

1 c. coarsely chopped broccoli florets
1 c. coarsely chopped cauliflower
1 c. shredded carrots
4 tbsp. sunflower seeds
1 11-oz. can mandarin oranges
   in juice, drained
2 tbsp. fat-free Miracle Whip
¼ c. buttermilk
2 packets artificial sweetener
2 tbsp. imitation bacon bits

3 large Granny Smith apples,
   cored and diced
½ c. raisins
1 c. chopped celery
½ c. walnuts
1 1.4-oz. box sugar-free butterscotch-
   flavored nonfat instant pudding
2 c. artificially sweetened plain
   nonfat yogurt

BROCCOLI-CAULIFLOWER SALAD

Contributed by Freda Virnau, Waco, Texas

Combine broccoli, cauliflower, carrots, sunflower seeds and mandarin oranges in medium bowl; set aside. In separate bowl, blend together Miracle Whip, buttermilk and sweetener; pour over vegetables. Top with bacon bits prior to serving. Serves 8.
Exchanges: 1 vegetable, ½ fruit, 1 fat

CARAMEL APPLE SALAD

Contributed by Patti McCoy, Fort Lupton, Colorado

In large bowl, combine apples, raisins, celery and walnuts; set aside. In small bowl combine pudding mix and yogurt; pour into apple mixture and stir to coat. Refrigerate at least 1 hour. Serves 6.
Exchanges: ½ meat, 1 fruit, ½ milk, 1 fat

SIDE DISHES

Salads, Slaws and Marinated Veggies

CHICKEN-SPINACH SALAD

Contributed by Adina Collins, New Orleans, Louisiana

Combine all ingredients in large salad bowl; toss to coat evenly. Serves 3.
Exchanges: 1 ½ meats, ½ vegetable, 1 fat

3 oz. cooked chicken breast,
   cooled and chopped
2 c. fresh spinach
½ large tomato, chopped
½ cucumber, chopped
¼ c. almonds
2 tbsp. balsamic vinegar

CHINESE COLESLAW

Contributed by Kay Smith, Roscoe, Texas

Crush ramen noodles and mix with seasoning packet provided with noodles in medium bowl. Add cabbage; mix well and refrigerate. Combine onion, almonds, sesame seeds, margarine, vinegar, Italian dressing, artificial sweetener and pepper in large jar with lid; shake well and pour over slaw just prior to serving. Serves 8.
Exchanges: ½ bread, 1 vegetable, ½ fat

8 c. shredded cabbage
1 3-oz. pkg. chicken-flavored low-fat
   ramen noodle soup
½ c. chopped green onion
1 oz. slivered almonds
1 tbsp. sesame seeds
1 tbsp. reduced-calorie margarine,
   melted
3 tbsp. rice vinegar
½ c. fat-free Italian dressing
2 packets artificial sweetener
¼ tsp. black pepper

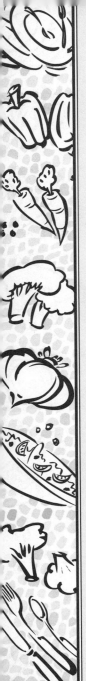

1   15½-oz. can kidney beans, rinsed
    and drained
1   15½-oz. can garbanzo beans,
    rinsed and drained
1   15-oz. can diced tomatoes, drained
    with 4 tbsp. liquid reserved
2½ c. diced green bell pepper
2   c. cauliflower flowerets, lightly
    steamed
2   c. broccoli florets, lightly steamed
2   c. diced zucchini
½   c. diced Vidalia onion
1½ c. peas (canned or frozen)
1½ c. corn (canned or frozen)
6   tbsp. red wine vinegar
1   tbsp. olive oil
2   tsp. Italian seasoning
2   tsp. garlic powder
2   tsp. salt
2   tsp. pepper

CONFETTI PARTY SALAD

*Contributed by Susan Bauman, Grand Island, New York,
and Diane Temple, Tonawan, New York*

Drain tomatoes, reserving 4 tablespoons of liquid; set aside. In large bowl, combine beans, tomatoes, bell pepper, cauliflower, broccoli, zucchini, onion, peas and corn; mix well and set aside. Combine reserved tomato juice, vinegar, oil, Italian seasoning, garlic powder, salt and pepper in small jar with lid; shake well and pour over salad, tossing gently to coat. Cover and refrigerate at least 4 hours. Serves 30.
Exchanges: ½ bread, ½ vegetable

Tip: This recipe is versatile! Here are some suggested variations:
- Add 12 ounces fat-free or low-fat provolone or mozzarella cheese just prior to serving. (Add ¾ meat exchange.)
- Add 24 ounces cooked diced chicken. (Add 1¼ meat exchanges.)
- Substitute an equal amount of Greek seasoning for the Italian seasoning and add 12 ounces crumbled feta cheese. (Add ¾ meat and ½ fat exchanges.)
- Serve with a 3-ounce grilled chicken breast and ½ warmed 6-inch pita. (Add 3¾ meats, ½ bread and ½ fat exchanges.)
- Make the salad dressing alone to use on other pasta or salad dishes. (The exchange for the dressing by itself is ½ fat per 2-tablespoon serving.)

CORNBREAD SALAD

Contributed by Jennifer Nelson, Little Rock, Mississippi

Cook cornbread according to directions on package; cool and crumble. Set aside. Combine mayonnaise, sour cream and ranch-dressing mix in medium bowl; mix well and set aside. Layer ingredients in 9x13-inch baking dish *in following order*: cornbread, beans, corn, dressing mixture, tomatoes, salt, pepper, onions, bell pepper, cheese and bacon pieces. Chill several hours or overnight before serving. Serves 12.

Exchanges: ½ meat, 1½ breads, ½ vegetable

1   6-oz. package Mexican-style cornbread mix
1   c. fat-free mayonnaise
1   8-oz. container fat-free sour cream
1   envelope ranch-style dressing mix
1   15-oz. can can dark red kidney beans, drained
1   15.2-oz. can corn, drained
4   tomatoes, peeled and diced
    Salt and pepper to taste
½   c. chopped green onions
½   c. chopped green bell pepper
2   c. shredded fat-free cheddar cheese
1   2-oz. jar reduced-fat Hormel Real Bacon pieces

COTTAGE SALAD

Contributed by Karen D. Jernigan, Thibodaux, Louisiana

In large bowl, combine all ingredients; toss well. Refrigerate 2 hours or until ready to serve. Serves 2.

Exchanges: ½ vegetable, 2 milks

1   16-oz. container low-fat cottage cheese
¼   c. diced red bell pepper
¼   c. diced green bell pepper
¼   c. diced green onion
¼   c. diced tomatoes
½   tsp. Italian seasoning

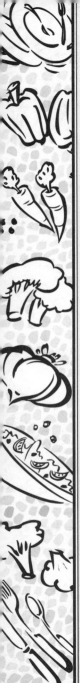

- 1 15-oz. can chunky mixed fruit in juice, drained
- 2 medium bananas, sliced
- 1 c. sliced strawberries
- ½ c. artificially sweetened lemon-flavored low-fat yogurt
- ½ c. fat-free whipped topping, thawed

- 1 large head green leaf lettuce, torn into bite-sized pieces
- 2 c. fresh strawberries
- 2 c. fresh blueberries
- 1 8-oz. can mandarin oranges in juice, drained
- 1 16-oz. can pineapple chunks in water, drained
- 2 tbsp. chopped pecans

CREAMY FRUIT SALAD

Contributed by Joe Ann Winkler, Overland Park, Kansas

Combine mixed fruit, bananas and strawberries in medium bowl. Gently fold in yogurt and whipped topping, until fruit is coated. Refrigerate until ready to serve. Serves 4.

Exchanges: 1 fruit

Tip: Although this recipe calls for lemon-flavored yogurt, you can experiment with other flavors to fit your taste buds!

EASY SUMMER SALAD

Contributed by Cheryl Shouse, Fairview, Pennsylvania

In large salad bowl, combine lettuce, strawberries, blueberries, mandarin oranges and pineapple chunks; toss and sprinkle with pecans. Serves 6.

Exchanges: 1 fruit, ⅓ fat

Tip: This is great without salad dressing, but you can serve it with 2 tablespoons of your favorite fat-free salad dressing, if desired. (This will not alter the exchanges.)

FRESH GARDEN SALAD

Contributed by Mary Russell, Basin, Wyoming

Combine tomatoes, cucumbers, avocados and onion in large salad bowl; mix well and toss with salad dressing. Let sit 15 to 30 minutes. Serves 26.
Exchanges: ½ vegetable, ½ fat

Tip: Serve this salad with 2 breadsticks per person for a light summertime meal! (Add 1 bread exchange.)

---

3 large tomatoes, coarsely chopped
3 large cucumbers, coarsely chopped
   (peel before chopping if skin is tough)
2 medium avocados, peeled, seeded
   and diced
1 large sweet onion, coarsely chopped
1 8-oz. bottle fat-free Wishbone
   Italian salad dressing

GRAPE SALAD

Contributed by Patsy Collins, Natchez, Mississippi

Sprinkle dry gelatin over ½ cup juice in shallow dish; set aside. Pour remaining juice into small saucepan and bring to gentle boil. Pour into dish with gelatin; stir until gelatin is dissolved. Stir in sweetener, grapes and pecans. Refrigerate until set, stirring several times during setting time to mix fruit and pecans equally. Serves 8.
Exchanges: 1 fruit, ½ fat

1 envelope plain gelatin
2 c. grape juice, divided
4 packets artificial sweetener
   (not aspartame)
¾ c. sliced grapes
¼ c. chopped pecans

MARINATED ITALIAN GREEN BEANS

Contributed by Lynda Martinaz, Madison, Mississippi

Combine green beans and onion in medium bowl. Add Italian dressing; toss gently to coat. Cover and refrigerate at least 30 minutes. Gently stir again just prior to serving. Serves 4.
Exchanges: 1 vegetable

1 15-oz. can Italian-style green
   beans, rinsed and drained
½ c. finely chopped onion
¼ c. fat-free Italian dressing

SIDE DISHES

Salads, Slaws and Marinated Veggies

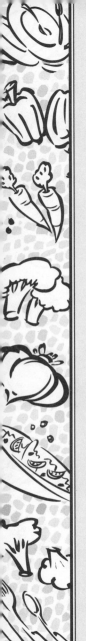

1   15-oz. can peas, drained (can sub-
    stitute black-eyed peas or green beans)
1   15-oz. can corn, drained
1   3-oz. can pimientos, drained
    and chopped
2   c. chopped celery
1½ c. chopped bell pepper
1   c. chopped onion
12 packets artificial sweetener
½   c. apple-cider vinegar
2   tsp. oil
¼   tbsp. salt

16 oz. penne rigate pasta
3   qts. water
4   chicken bouillon cubes
1   tbsp. seasoned salt
1   green bell pepper, thinly sliced
1   red bell pepper, thinly sliced
1   yellow bell pepper, thinly sliced
8   oz. mushrooms, thinly sliced
12 black olives, thinly sliced
1   bunch green onions, tops only,
    chopped
1   8-oz. bottle fat-free salad dressing

MARINATED VEGETABLES

Contributed by Georgia Senn, Gilmer, Texas

Combine peas, corn, pimientos, celery, bell pepper and onion in large bowl; set aside. In small bowl, combine sweetener, vinegar, oil and salt; stir well and pour over vegetables. Stir well to coat; marinate overnight in refrigerator. Serves 8.
Exchanges: 1 bread, ½ vegetable, ½ fat

Tip: This dish will keep in your refrigerator for several days!

PASTA SALAD

Contributed by Lisa Cramer, Houston, Texas

In large saucepan, bring water, bouillon and seasoned salt to boil. Add pasta and boil until tender. Drain liquid; add bell peppers, mushrooms, olives and green onions; toss to mix. Pour dressing over pasta; toss again to coat. Refrigerate until ready to serve. Serves 12.
Exchanges: 2 breads, ½ vegetable

Tip: To make a meal, top each serving with one of the following:
- 2 ounces grilled chicken (Add 2 meat exchanges.)
- 2 ounces shrimp (Add 1 meat exchange.)
- 2 ounces tuna (Add 1 meat exchange.)

PEARL'S TUNA SALAD

Contributed by Pauline Hines, New Orleans, Louisiana

Combine tuna, egg whites, pickle, celery, bell pepper, onion, green onions, mayonnaise, mustard, seasoned salt, black pepper, cayenne pepper, parsley and paprika in large bowl; mix well. Cover and chill. When ready to serve, garnish with egg ring in the center and sprinkle entire salad with light dusting of paprika. Serves 6.
Exchanges: 1 ½ meats, ½ vegetable

2	6-oz. cans tuna in water, drained
2	hard-boiled egg whites, diced
½	c. chopped dill pickle
½	c. chopped celery
½	c. chopped green bell pepper
½	c. minced onion
½	c. chopped green onions
2	tbsp. low-fat mayonnaise
1	tbsp. mustard
¼	tsp. seasoned salt
2	tsp. ground black pepper
¼	tsp. cayenne pepper
2	tbsp. parsley
1	tbsp. paprika
1	hard-boiled egg ring for garnish

PINEAPPLE GELATIN SALAD

Contributed by Lisa Cramer, Houston, Texas

Prepare gelatin according to package directions; set aside. Spoon equal amount of pineapple into each of 10 dessert dishes. Pour gelatin mixture over pineapple and refrigerate 1 hour or until set. Top each with dollop of whipped topping prior to serving. Serves 10.
Exchanges: ½ fruit

1	20-oz. can crushed pineapple in juice, drained
2	.3-oz. boxes sugar-free gelatin (any flavor)
2	c. fat-free whipped topping

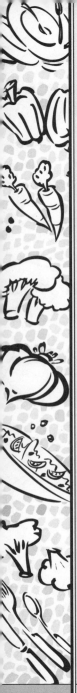

- 1 envelope plain gelatin
- 2 c. pineapple juice, divided
- 1 11-oz. can crushed pineapple in juice, drained
- 1 8-oz. can mandarin oranges in juice, drained
- 4 packets artificial sweetener (not aspartame)

- 2 c. coleslaw mix (can use shredded fresh red or green cabbage)
- 1 c. grated carrots
- 1 11-oz. can mandarin oranges in juice, rinsed and drained
- 2 tbsp. chopped pecans
- ¼ c. low-fat mayonnaise
- 2 tbsp. sugar-free maple syrup

PINEAPPLE-ORANGE SALAD

Contributed by Patsy Collins, Natchez, Mississippi

Sprinkle dry gelatin over ½ cup pineapple juice in shallow dish; set aside. Pour remaining juice into small saucepan and bring to gentle boil. Pour into dish with gelatin; stir until gelatin is dissolved. Add pineapple, oranges and sweetener. Refrigerate 1 hour or until set. Serves 6.

Exchanges: 1 ½ fruits

SOUTHERN BELLE COLESLAW

Contributed by Lynda Martinaz, Madison, Mississippi

In large bowl, combine coleslaw mix (or cabbage), carrots, oranges and pecans; mix well and set aside. In small bowl, blend together mayonnaise and syrup; add to coleslaw mixture and toss gently to combine. Cover and refrigerate at least 30 minutes. Gently stir again before serving. Serves 4.

Exchanges: 1 vegetable, ½ fruit, 1 fat

SOUTHWEST-STYLE POTATO SALAD

Contributed by Joyce Pillitteri, Jacksonville, Florida

Combine yogurt, mayonnaise, lemon juice, cumin and coriander in large bowl. Salt and pepper to taste; add potato cubes, onion, celery, minced poblano and jalapeño peppers, olives and cilantro. Mix well. Refrigerate until ready to serve. Serves 12.
Exchanges: ½ bread, ½ vegetable, ½ fat

6	large red potatoes, cooked, cooled and cubed
½	c. plain nonfat yogurt
½	c. low-fat mayonnaise
2	tbsp. lemon juice
1	tsp. cumin
½	tsp. coriander
	Salt and pepper to taste
1	small red onion, finely diced
3	celery stalks, finely diced
1	poblano pepper, minced
2	pickled jalapeño peppers, minced
10	green Spanish olives with pimiento, thinly sliced
2	tbsp. finely chopped cilantro

SPINACH SALAD

Contributed by Becky Toney, Tarpon Springs, Florida

In small bowl, mash egg yolks with fork; add mustard, vinegar and sugar substitute. Mix well and set aside. In separate bowl, chop egg whites; set aside. Cut or tear spinach into bite-sized pieces; arrange in large salad bowl and toss with egg-yolk dressing. Top with egg whites and onions. Serve immediately. Serves 6.
Exchanges: ½ meat, 2½ vegetables, ½ fat

2	c. fresh spinach, washed and dried
3	eggs, hard-boiled, whites and yolks separated
1½	tsp. prepared yellow mustard
3	tbsp. apple-cider vinegar
3	tbsp. sugar substitute
2	green onions, thinly sliced

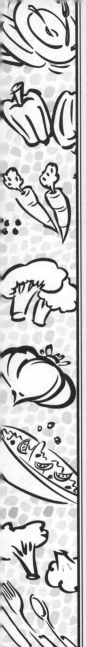

1 20-oz. can pineapple chunks,
   drained with ½ c. juice reserved
6 c. chopped red apples
1½ c. chopped celery
½ c. raisins
¼ c. soy nuts
½ c. fat-free mayonnaise
½ c. plain nonfat yogurt
2 tbsp. sugar substitute

1 c. uncooked shrimp, shelled
   and deveined
2 c. whole-wheat spiral pasta, cooked
   and drained
1½ tbsp. vegetable oil
½ c. chopped red onion
1½ tbsp. vinegar
½ c. chopped red bell pepper
½ c. chopped green bell pepper
½ c. chopped yellow bell pepper

WALDORF SALAD

Contributed by Kathi Reinecke, Riverview, Florida

Drain pineapple, reserving ½ cup juice. Combine pineapple, apples, celery, raisins and soy nuts in large bowl; set aside. In separate bowl, blend reserved pineapple juice, mayonnaise, yogurt and sugar substitute; add to fruit mixture and toss until well coated. Chill 2 hours and serve. Serves 16.
Exchanges: 1 fruit

WHOLE-WHEAT SPIRALS SALAD

Contributed by Eloria Phipps, New Orleans, Louisiana

In nonstick skillet over medium-high heat, sauté shrimp in oil until pink in color; season to taste. Combine shrimp, pasta, onion, vinegar and bell peppers in large serving bowl; mix well. Serves 8.
Exchanges: 1 meat, 1½ breads, ½ vegetable, ½ fat

SOUPS

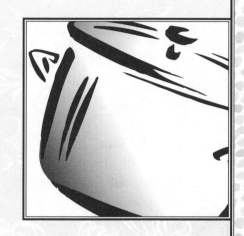

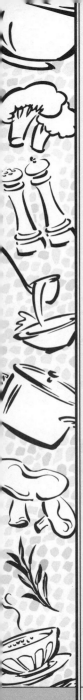

Soups

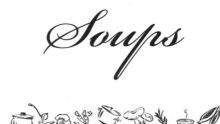

BUTTERNUT SQUASH SOUP

Contributed by Cory Beckman, Vacaville, California

1 2-lb. butternut squash, sliced in half lengthwise
10 fresh sage leaves
2 c. chopped onion
1 leek, minced, white only
2 Granny Smith apples, peeled and chopped
4 c. chicken broth
Salt to taste
Nonstick cooking spray

Place 5 sage leaves on each half of squash; cover halves with plastic wrap and microwave on high, rotating every 3 minutes, until soft. Remove sage; discard. Remove seeds; discard. Scoop out squash; set aside. Over medium heat, in large pot coated with cooking spray, sauté onion, leek and apples until tender. Add squash and cover with chicken broth. Pour mixture into blender to ¾ full. Very carefully puree. Pour the pureed soup into large bowl; repeat until all soup has been pureed and then pour back into soup pot. Keep warm until ready to serve. Serves 8.

Exchanges: ½ **bread,** ½ **vegetable,** ½ **fruit**

Tip: This soup is very filling, but you can add 16 ounces chopped cooked chicken for even more substance. (Add 2 meat exchanges.)

CHEDDAR CHEESE SOUP

Contributed by Johnny Lewis, San Leon, Texas

In medium saucepan, bring water, carrots, celery and green onions to boil; allow to boil 5 minutes; remove from heat and set aside. Sauté white onion in skillet with margarine; stir in flour, blending well. Remove from heat and set aside. Bring milk and chicken broth to boil in small saucepan; stir briskly into white-onion mixture using wire whisk. Add cheese, salt, pepper and cayenne; stir well. Add mustard and boiled vegetables, including water; stir well and bring to boil. Serve immediately. (Do not blend in food processor.) Serves 16.

Exchanges: ½ meat, ¼ bread, ½ milk, 1 ½ fats

15	oz. Cheez Whiz Light
2	c. water
½	c. finely chopped carrots
1	c. finely chopped celery
1	c. finely chopped green onions
1	medium white onion, chopped
2	tbsp. reduced-calorie margarine
1	c. flour
4	c. nonfat milk
4	c. chicken broth
	Salt and pepper to taste
¼	tsp. cayenne pepper
1	tbsp. prepared mustard

ITALIAN GARDEN SOUP

Contributed by Lynda Martinaz, Madison, Mississippi

Combine all ingredients in large pot; cook over medium-high heat until heated through. Serves 14.

Exchanges: ½ meat, 1 ½ vegetables

> **Tip:** This is a great Crock-Pot dish! Just add the ingredients and set the cooking temperature to low—in 3 hours you'll have a wonderful soup!

1	15-oz. can Italian-style cut green beans
1	15-oz. can Italian-style stewed tomatoes
1	8-oz. can tomato sauce, with basil, garlic and oregano
1	14 ½-oz. can zucchini with tomatoes
1	15-oz. can peas and carrots
1	6-oz. can chunk white chicken in water
3	15-oz. cans fat-free chicken broth

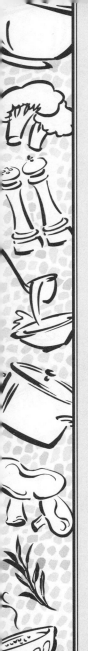

1 lb. boneless, skinless chicken breasts
3 qts. water
8 oz. tomato sauce
10 chicken bouillon cubes
4 c. cubed potatoes
3 c. sliced carrots, ½ in. thick
3 c. cubed zucchini
2 c. coarsely chopped onion
2 c. corn (fresh or frozen)
3 c. green beans (fresh or frozen)

1 lb. lean ground beef
2 tsp. olive oil
2 large onions, chopped
2 c. diced carrots
2 c. diced celery
3 c. diced zucchini
½ c. granulated beef bouillon
6 c. water, divided
2 tsp. dried oregano
1 tsp. black pepper
3 tbsp. parsley
2 tsp. hot pepper sauce
6 c. chunky pasta sauce
1 15-oz. can red kidney beans,
  drained and rinsed
1 19-oz. can white kidney beans,
  drained and rinsed
2 c. cooked macaroni or small pasta
  shells

SOUPS

MEGA-CHICKEN VEGETABLE SOUP

Contributed by Johnny Lewis, San Leon, Texas

In large pot, boil chicken breasts with water until cooked through. Remove breasts and set aside to cool. Add tomato sauce, bouillon, potatoes, carrots, zucchini, onion, corn and green beans to broth; bring to slow boil. Cook 45 minutes or until vegetables are firm but done. Cut breasts into bite-sized pieces; add to soup. Serves 12.
Exchanges: 1½ meats, 1 bread, 1 vegetable

PASTA E FAGIOLI

Contributed by Becky Sirt, The Woodlands, Texas

In preheated soup pot, brown ground beef with olive oil over medium-high heat, stirring constantly to break up. Add onion, carrots, celery and zucchini; sauté 10 minutes more and reduce heat to simmer. Dissolve beef bouillon in small bowl with 1 cup hot water; stir in oregano, black pepper, parsley and hot pepper sauce. Add mixture to beef; stir in pasta sauce. Simmer 10 minutes; stir in remaining 5 cups water (or enough to reach desired consistency). Stir and simmer 30 minutes more. Add beans and pasta just prior to serving. Serves 16.
Exchanges: 1 meat, 1½ breads, 1 vegetable, ½ fat

SAVORY POTATO SOUP

Contributed by Miriam Rust, Charlotte, North Carolina

Put potatoes, celery, onion, salt and pepper in soup pot; add just enough water to cover potatoes and cook until potatoes are tender. Melt margarine in skillet; add flour and dill, mixing well. Add milk gradually, stirring constantly to make smooth sauce. Cook 5 minutes; add drained vegetable mixture and heat thoroughly. Serves 6.

Exchanges: 1 bread, ½ milk, 1 fat

3	c. peeled, diced potatoes
1	c. chopped celery
½	c. chopped onion
1	tsp. salt
¼	tsp. pepper
2	tbsp. margarine
2	tbsp. flour
1	tsp. dill
3	c. nonfat milk

SMOKED-SAUSAGE AND POTATO SOUP

Contributed by Ronda Robbs, Fredericktown, Missouri

Combine sausages, potatoes, onion, carrot, parsley, garlic, chicken broth, water, salt and pepper in large pot. Bring to boil; cover and simmer 15 to 20 minutes or until potatoes are tender. Place flour in small bowl; slowly add milk, stirring constantly with wire whisk to prevent lumps. Pour mixture into soup, stirring constantly. Bring to boil until heated through. Serves 8.

Exchanges: 1½ meats, 1 bread

- -

Tip: For added fiber, don't peel potatoes before cutting into cubes

14	oz. lean smoked-turkey sausages, cubed
5	potatoes, peeled and cubed
½	c. chopped onion
¼	c. grated carrot
1	tbsp. chopped fresh parsley (or ½ tsp. dried)
½	tsp. crushed garlic
2	14½-oz. cans chicken broth
4½	c. water
1	tsp. salt
¼	tsp. pepper
⅓	c. flour
1	c. nonfat milk

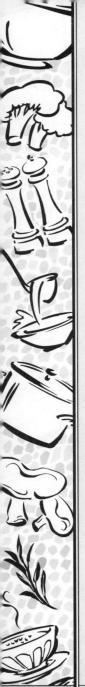

2 c. chicken, cooked and shredded
4 14-oz. cans fat-free chicken broth
1 c. peeled, sliced carrots
1 c. snow peas, cut diagonally into strips
¼ c. instant rice
2 scallions, sliced
Salt and pepper to taste

16 oz. extra-lean ground beef
1 c. chopped onion
4 beef bouillon cubes
2 tbsp. water
2½ c. sliced carrots
3 c. pinto beans, thoroughly rinsed and drained
2 c. corn, drained
3 c. peeled and diced red potatoes
1 envelope taco seasoning mix
1 envelope ranch-style dressing mix
1¼ c. Rotel tomatoes with green chiles
8 c. water

SPEEDY CHICKEN SOUP
Contributed by Joy Jarvis, Norcross, Georgia

Bring broth to boil in large pot over high heat; add chicken, carrots, snow peas, rice and scallions. Reduce heat and simmer 5 minutes more or until carrots are tender. Season with salt and pepper. Serve immediately or allow to cool and freeze for later use. Serves 4.
Exchanges: 4 meats, 1 bread, 1 vegetable, 1 fat

TACO SOUP
Contributed by Johnny Lewis, San Leon, Texas

Lightly brown ground beef in large skillet. Remove from skillet; drain and rinse with hot water and set aside. Use same skillet to lightly sauté onion and bouillon cubes in 2 tablespoons water. Return meat to skillet; add carrots, beans, corn, red potatoes, taco seasoning, ranch dressing mix, tomatoes and water. Bring to boil and simmer 20 to 30 minutes. Serves 10.
Exchanges: 1½ meats, 1½ breads, 1 vegetable

Tip: For a variety, try the following substitutions (none of which will alter the exchanges):
- Use 6 ounces chicken breasts or 6 ounces extra-lean ground turkey instead of ground beef. (If chicken is substituted, use chicken bouillon cubes instead of beef bouillion cubes.)
- Use 1¼ cups stewed tomatoes instead of Rotel tomatoes.
- Use 2 cups hominy instead of corn.
- Add up to 2 jalapeño peppers to add a hot and spicy taste!

WHITE BEAN SOUP

Contributed by Johnny Lewis, San Leon, Texas

Put beans in large pot; cover with water. Add bouillon cubes, garlic, seasoned salt and onion; boil gently 1 ½ hours or until beans are almost tender. Add carrots and celery; continue cooking until tender. Add corn and cook 8 minutes more. (Note: If extra water is needed while beans are cooking, bring water to boil before adding to beans.) Serves 8.

Exchanges: 1 bread

1   lb. navy beans
4   chicken bouillon cubes
4   garlic cloves
    Seasoned salt to taste
1   onion, finely chopped
1   c. chopped carrots
1   c. chopped celery
1   c. corn (fresh or frozen)

THIS 'N' THAT

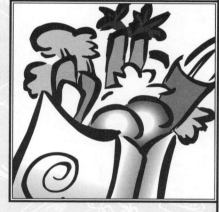

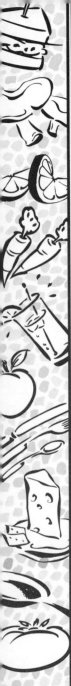

1 c. dried apricots
1 c. unsweetened apple juice

This 'n' That

DIPS AND SPREADS

APRICOT SPREAD

Contributed by Lynda Martinaz, Madison, Mississippi

Combine apricots and apple juice in small saucepan; bring to boil over medium-high heat. Reduce heat to low; cover and simmer 20 minutes, stirring occasionally. Remove from heat. Allow to cool slightly; pour cooled mixture into blender or food processor and blend until smooth. Finish cooling to room temperature and refrigerate in airtight container or jar with tight fitting lid up to 3 months. Serves 16.
Exchanges: ½ **fruit**

BEST FRIEND'S CUCUMBER DIP

Contributed by Judy Marshall, Gilmer, Texas

Use grating blade in food processor to grate cucumber; press with paper towel to remove excess liquid. Replace grating blade with cutting blade; add radishes, bell pepper and onions. Mix quickly, but do not liquefy. Drain excess liquid. Add sour cream, Miracle Whip, chile sauce, garlic, cayenne pepper, dill weed, parsley and salt. Mix well by hand; chill and serve with fresh vegetables or baked chips or crackers. Serves 16.
Exchanges: Free

1 cucumber
½ bunch (approximately 3 oz.) medium-sized radishes
½ green bell pepper
½ c. chopped green onions, tops included
1 c. fat-free sour cream
½ c. fat-free Miracle Whip
3 tbsp. chile sauce
¼ tsp. minced garlic
   Dash cayenne pepper
   (or red pepper sauce)
½ tsp. crushed dried dill weed
1 tsp. crushed dried parsley
½ tsp. salt

CHEESE DIP

Contributed by Martha Rogers, Houston, Texas

Place cheese and tomatoes in microwave-safe bowl and microwave on high 1 minute. Stir and continue heating at 1-minute intervals until completely melted. Serves 6.
Exchanges: 1 ½ meats, ½ bread

1 8-oz. jar Cheese Whiz Light
½ 10-oz. can Rotel tomatoes

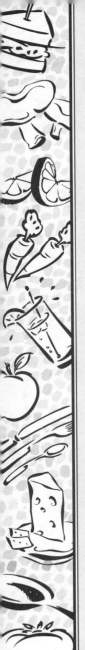

1 8-oz. pkg. fat-free cream cheese
¼ c. Nesquik no-sugar added
   chocolate-flavored drink mix
⅛ c. decaffeinated coffee
½ tsp. coconut extract
1 packet artificial sweetener
½ c. fat-free whipped topping

1 16-oz. container artificially
   sweetened lemon-flavored low-fat
   yogurt
1 8-oz. pkg. fat-free cream cheese

1 8-oz. pkg. fat-free cream cheese,
   softened
1 14-oz. jar pizza sauce
2 c. grated mozzarella cheese
4 oz. chopped black olives
1 4.2-oz. pkg. chopped soy pepperoni

CHOCOLATE FRUIT DIP
Contributed by Lynda Martinaz, Madison, Mississippi

In a medium bowl, stir cream cheese with a spoon until soft. Add chocolate drink mix, coffee, coconut extract and sweetener; mix well. Blend in whipped topping; refrigerate at least 1 hour. Gently stir again prior to serving. Serves 8.
Exchanges: ½ meat, ½ bread

FRUIT DIP
Contributed by Martha Rogers, Houston, Texas

Combine yogurt and cream cheese in small bowl; blend together. Refrigerate 30 minutes. Serves 8.
Exchanges: ½ meat

PIZZA DIP
Contributed by Diana Robinson, Lithonia, Georgia

Preheat oven to 350° F. Spread cream cheese in bottom of glass pie or quiche pan. Layer pizza sauce over cream cheese; then add remaining ingredients *in following order:* cheese, olives and pepperoni. Bake 25 minutes; serve warm. Serves 8.
Exchanges: 1 ½ meats, ½ vegetable, 1 fat

THIS 'N' THAT

Dips and Spreads

QUICK BEAN DIP

Contributed by Sandra Vigil, Platteville, Colorado

Mix beans and salsa in small bowl; season to taste. Serves 4.
Exchanges: 1 ½ breads, ½ vegetable

1   16-oz. can fat-free refried beans
½   c. salsa (any kind)
    Salt and pepper to taste
    Other seasonings of your
    choice to taste

SHRIMP DIP

Contributed by Daisy O. Mixon, Columbia, South Carolina

Mix cream cheese, mayonnaise, ketchup and shrimp; refrigerate until 15 minutes prior to serving. Serves 4.
Exchanges: 2 meats, ½ bread

4 ¼   oz. canned shrimp, coarsely
     chopped
1   8-oz. pkg. fat-free cream cheese,
    softened
¼   c. fat-free mayonnaise
1   tbsp. ketchup

SPINACH AND ARTICHOKE SPREAD

Contributed by John Montieth, Greeley, Colorado

With blade running in food processor, drop in garlic cloves to mince. Add artichoke hearts and spinach; pulse-process until all are finely chopped, scraping bowl often. In a medium bowl, combine cream cheese, salt, seasoned pepper, onion and lemon pepper; blend well. Add contents of food processor and mix to combine. Refrigerate at least 1 hour. Serves 8.
Exchanges: 1 meat, 1 vegetable

1   14-oz. can artichoke hearts,
    drained and quartered
1   10-oz. pkg. frozen chopped
    spinach, thawed and well drained
2   cloves garlic, peeled
1   8-oz. pkg. fat-free cream cheese,
    softened
1   tsp. seasoned salt
½   tsp. seasoned pepper
1   tbsp. prepared minced onion
1   tsp. lemon pepper

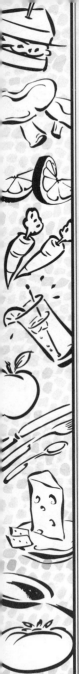

1 10-oz. pkg. frozen chopped
   spinach, thawed and well drained
1 c. fat-free Miracle Whip
1 c. fat-free sour cream
1 tbsp. minced onion
1 envelope vegetable soup mix

4 chicken bouillon cubes
3 c. water
2 tbsp. flour
   Salt and pepper to taste

SPINACH DIP
Contributed by Martha Rogers, Houston, Texas

Combine all ingredients in a small bowl. Refrigerate overnight to allow flavors to blend. Serves 6.
Exchanges: ½ meat, ½ bread, ½ vegetable

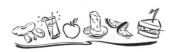

GRAVY AND SAUCES

GRAVY FOR CORNBREAD DRESSING
Contributed by Johnny Lewis, San Leon, Texas

Add bouillon to water boiling in large saucepan. In a pint jar with lid, combine ¾ cup of bouillon water with flour; shake well. Slowly pour into remaining water, stirring constantly to prevent lumps. Simmer over low heat, stirring frequently until gravy consistency is reached. Add flour or water if needed to reach desired consistency. Add salt and pepper to taste. Serves 16.
Exchanges: Free

PASTA SAUCE

Contributed by Johnny Lewis, San Leon, Texas

In a saucepan combine water, basil, oregano and bouillon; bring to a boil and let steep 3 to 5 minutes. Pour through tea strainer; discard solids and return liquid to saucepan. Add tomatoes, tomato paste, onion, garlic and pepper; simmer uncovered 45 minutes or until thickened. Serves 6.

Exchanges: ½ bread, 1 vegetable

2 c. water
4 tbsp. basil
2 tbsp. oregano
8 chicken bouillon cubes
1 29-oz. can tomatoes, crushed
6 oz. tomato paste
1 ½ c. finely chopped onion
8 garlic cloves, crushed
½ tsp. cayenne pepper

Tip: Sauces can be served on pasta, meat or vegetables, depending on your taste. Here are some suggestions and the exchanges to add:
- ½ cup cooked pasta (Add 1 bread exchange.)
- 2 ounces sliced grilled chicken (Add 2 meat exchanges.)
- ½ cup steamed mixed vegetables (Add 1 vegetable exchange.)

PIZZA SAUCE

Contributed by Johnny Lewis, San Leon, Texas

Combine water, basil and oregano in saucepan; bring to boil and let steep 3 to 5 minutes. Stir in tomato sauce and tomato paste; simmer until desired consistency. Serves 12.

Exchanges: 1 vegetable

1 ½ c. water
1 tbsp. basil
½ tbsp. oregano
1 12-oz. can tomato sauce
1 6-oz. can tomato paste

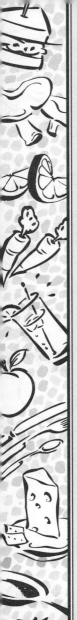

¼ c. brown-sugar substitute
1 tbsp. cornstarch
⅓ c. lemon juice
⅓ c. low-sodium soy sauce
⅓ c. water
1 tsp. minced onion
2 tbsp. reduced-calorie margarine
1 tsp. garlic powder

1 8-oz. bottle fat-free Italian salad dressing
2 tbsp. balsamic vinegar
1½ tbsp. dried basil

SOY-LEMON BASTING SAUCE

Contributed by Alyce Amussen, Silver Spring, Maryland

In small saucepan, combine brown-sugar substitute and cornstarch. Stir in lemon juice, soy sauce and water; mix thoroughly until smooth. Add onion, margarine and garlic powder; cook over medium heat until thickened and bubbly. Use to baste poultry, pork or fish during the last 15 minutes of grilling. Serves 4.
Exchanges: ½ fat

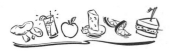

SALAD DRESSINGS

FAT-FREE ITALIAN DRESSING

Contributed by Johnny Lewis, San Leon, Texas

Combine all ingredients in container with lid; shake well to mix thoroughly. Refrigerate until ready to serve.
Exchanges: Free

Tip: This dressing will last up to 6 months in your refrigerator!

RASPBERRY VINAIGRETTE DRESSING

Contributed by Lisa Cramer, Houston, Texas

Combine all ingredients in small bowl; blend well and refrigerate. Serves 8.
Exchanges: Free

½ c. rice vinegar

⅓ c. seedless raspberry all-fruit spread

2 tbsp. applesauce

2 tbsp. chopped pecans

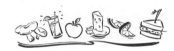

MISCELLANEOUS

BREAD-PUDDING BREAKFAST DISH

Contributed by Carol Glaman, Fond du Lac, Wisconsin

In a microwave-safe bowl, combine egg whites, milk, vanilla and sugar substitute;
fold in bread chunks and raisins and microwave on high 3 minutes. Serves 1.
Exchanges: 1 bread, 1 meat, ½ fruit and ½ milk

2 egg whites

½ c. nonfat milk

1 tsp. vanilla

2 tsp. sugar substitute

1 slice Texas-style bread, broken
into chunks

1 tsp. raisins

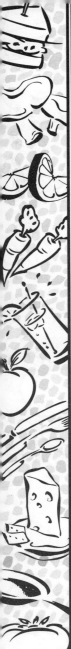

1 ½ c. flour
½ tsp. salt
3 tbsp. shortening
1 egg, well beaten
5 tbsp. water or chicken broth

OLD-FASHIONED STRIP DUMPLINGS

Contributed by Peggy Grooms, Sherman, Texas

Mix flour, salt, shortening and egg to form soft dough; divide into 3 parts. Roll out very thick and let dry 20 minutes. Cut into thin strips; drop into hot water or chicken broth and simmer until done. Serves 6.

Exchanges: 1 ½ breads, 1 ½ fats

Tip: Add 12 ounces cut up cooked chicken breasts to make chicken and dumplings. (Add 2 meat exchanges.)

Contributors

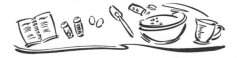

Donna Alley
Oxford, Nova Scotia, Canada

Alyce Amussen
Silver Spring, Maryland

Julie Anderson
Holland, Michigan

Margaret Anderson
Houston, Texas

Connie Armstrong
Hattiesburg, Mississippi

Evelyn Bailey
New Orleans, Louisiana

Barbara Bartlett
Kensington, Maryland

Susan Bauman
Grand Island, New York

Janet Bayless
Clinton, Tennessee

Cory Beckman
Vacaville, California

Irene Bell
Aynor, South Carolina

Julie Blackburn
Camden, Tennessee

Tammie Bogin
Hendersonville, North Carolina

Inez Boudreaux
Scott, Louisiana

Stacy Bowden
Gilmer, Texas

Gretchen Brown
Forest Grove, Oregon

Sandy Bundick
Hitchcock, Texas

June Chapko
San Antonio, Texas

Stephanie Cheves
Houston, Texas

Anita Clayton
Lenoir City, Tennessee

Adina Collins
New Orleans, Louisiana

Patsy Collins
Natchez, Mississippi

Beth Cosby
Lexington, South Carolina

Lisa Cramer
Houston, Texas

Cyndi Crosby
Charlotte, North Carolina

Pam Danford
Ashford, Alabama

Ouida Donald
Louisville, Mississippi

Ann Ellis
Louisville, Mississippi

Julia Faulk
Louisville, Mississippi

Kelly Fisher
Houston, Texas

Susan Gehrum
Turbotville, Pennsylvania

Carol Glaman
Fond du Lac, Wisconsin

Blanche Gray
Huntsville, Alabama
Peggy Grooms
Sherman, Texas
Laura Hartness
Kernersville, North Carolina
Pauline Hines
New Orleans, Louisiana
Shirlene Hoke
Dallas, North Carolina
Carolyn Holmes
Zwolle, Louisiana
Ann Hornbeak
Houston, Texas
Melba S. Hudson
Orange, Texas
Ann Hykin
Clearwater, Florida
Karen Israel
Pensacola, Florida
Kathy Israel
Pensacola, Florida
Sheri Jackson
Okmulgee, Oklahoma
Jan Jarrett
Hendersonville, North Carolina
Joy Jarvis
Norcross, Georgia
Karen D. Jernigan
Thibodaux, Louisiana
Janet Kirkhart
Mount Orab, Ohio
Robbie Kribell
Buena Park, California
Johnny Lewis
San Leon, Texas
Beverly Lowe
Tampa, Florida
Joyce Luke
Meridian, Mississippi

Judy Marshall
Gilmer, Texas
Lynda Martinaz
Madison, Mississippi
Patti McCoy
Fort Lupton, Colorado
Kelly McQueen
Gilmer, Texas
Cheryl Milligan
Tracy, California
Daisy O. Mixon
Columbia, South Carolina
Vicki Mobley
Loganville, Georgia
John Montieth
Greeley, Colorado
Carol Moore
Meridian, Mississippi
Jennifer Nelson
Little Rock, Mississippi
Martha Norsworthy
Murray, Kentucky
Carolyn Owen
Charlotte Court House, Virginia
Eloria Phipps
New Orleans, Louisiana
Joyce Pillitteri
Jacksonville, Florida
Dick Porter
Hartsville, South Carolina
Elizabeth Price
Gaffney, South Carolina
Geneva Reed
Camden, Tennessee
Terri Reed
Monroe, Washington
Kathi Reinecke
Riverview, Florida
Curtis Reuben
New Orleans, Louisiana

Megan Riley
  Southport, Florida
Sheila Robbins
  Houston, Texas
Ronda Robbs
  Fredericktown, Missouri
Diana Robinson
  Lithonia, Georgia
Melba Rodgers
  Duck Hill, Mississippi
Martha Rogers
  Houston, Texas
Mary Russell
  Basin, Wyoming
Miriam Rust
  Charlotte, North Carolina
Georgia Senn
  Gilmer, Texas
Katina Shelby
  New Orleans, Louisiana
Tiffany Short
  Corpus Christi, Texas
Cheryl Shouse
  Fairview, Pennsylvania
Becky Sirt
  The Woodlands, Texas
Irene Sisk
  Coal Hill, Arkansas
Kay Smith
  Roscoe, Texas
Favi Sotelo
  Artesia, New Mexico

Brenda Starry
  Piedmont, Oklahoma
Tamara Taber
  Orangeville, California
Nancy Taylor
  Houston, Texas
Diane Temple
  Tonawan, New York
Twila Tillman
  Trenton, Missouri
Becky Toney
  Tarpon Springs, Florida
Mildred Trail
  Keswick, Virginia
Debbie Vanlandingham
  Ovilla, Texas
Frances Ventress
  New Orleans, Louisiana
Sandra Vigil
  Platteville, Colorado
Freda Virnau
  Waco, Texas
Patricia Welker
  Farmington, Illinois
Joe Ann Winkler
  Overland Park, Kansas
Sara Wollitz
  Callahan, Florida
Shelly Wright
  Colorado Springs, Colorado

Index

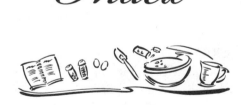

1-2-3 Easy Rolls, 38
Anytime Chocolate Latte, 54

ALFREDO SAUCE
Gilmont Chicken with, 123

APPETIZERS
No-Yolk Deviled Eggs, 32
Party Sandwich, 33
Pineapple Cheese Ball, 33
Simple Veggie Tortillas, 34
Spinach Wraps, 34
Tortilla Roll-Ups, 34
Vegetarian Quesadillas, 35
Apple Cobbler, 76
Apple Crisp, 76
Apple Dessert, 77
Apple Salad Mold, 71
Apple-Carrot Muffins, 40
Apple-Raisin Muffins, 40

APPLES, APPLESAUCE
Apple-Raisin Muffins, 40
Baked, 77
Caramel Salad, 144
Carrot Muffins, 40

Cobbler, 76
Crisp, 76
Dessert, 77
Oatmeal Pancakes, 50
Pie-Pan Tart, 64
Salad Mold, 71
Sugar-Free Applesauce Cake, 66
Sugar-Free Pie, 66
Sweet Potato Casserole, 142
Three-Layer Raisin Pie, 67
Apricot Spread, 164

ARTICHOKE
Spinach Spread, 167
Aunt Lottie's Crock-Pot Enchiladas, 86

ASPARAGUS
Peas and, 139
Baked Apples, 77
Baked Stuffed Fish, 99
Baked Tomatoes, 132
Baking Powder Biscuits, 38

BALSAMIC VINEGAR
Chicken with Rosemary, 111
Garlic Chicken Fillets in, 122
Balsamic Chicken with Rosemary, 111
Banana Bread, 45
Banana Milk Shake, 54
Banana Muffins, 41
Banana-Berry Smoothie, 55

BANANAS
Berry Cream Pie, 58
Berry Smoothie, 55
Bread, 45
Chocolate Cream Pie, 60
First Place Pudding, 73
Frozen Pineapple Cups, 69
Milk Shake, 54
Muffins, 41
Rich and Creamy Pudding, 75
Split Dessert, 77
Banana-Split Dessert, 77

BARBECUE
Chicken Kabobs, 111
Spoonburgers, 94

Turkey, 129
Barbecue Chicken Kabobs, 111

BARS
Breakfast, 46
Chewy Fruit-and-Oatmeal, 47
Light and Luscious Orange, 70
Oatmeal-Pecan, 81

BASIL
Lemon Carrots, 136

BASTING SAUCE
Soy-Lemon, 170

BEANS
Marinated Italian Green Beans, 149
Pasta e Fagioli, 158
Pinto á la Juan, 140
Quick Dip, 167
Superb Chili, 96
White Bean Soup, 161

BEEF
Aunt Lottie's Crock-Pot Enchiladas, 86
Cabbage Jambalaya, 87
Cajun Meat Loaf, 87
Easy Stew, 88
Green-Pepper Steak, 89
Jamie's Mexican Lasagna, 90
Light Mexican Manicotti, 91
Mexican-Style Venison Torte, 92
Shepherd's Pie, 93
Spaghetti Deluxe, 93
Spicy Swiss Steak, 94
Spoonburgers Barbecue, 94
Stay-Slim Lasagna, 95

Superb Chili and Beans, 96
Swedish Meatballs, 96
Tamale Pie, 97
Teague Tortilla Bake, 98
Beet Salad, 143

BERRY
Banana Cream Pie, 58
Banana Smoothie, 55
Very Berry Blueberry Muffins, 44
Best Friend's Cucumber Dip, 165

BEVERAGES
Anytime Chocolate Latte, 54
Banana Milk Shake, 54
Banana-Berry Smoothie, 55
Cappuccino Mix, 55
Cranberry Punch, 55
Quick and Easy Vanilla Malt, 56
Quick Cranberry Punch, 56
Strawberry Smoothie, 56
Tutti-Frutti Smoothie, 57
Wassail, 57

BISCUITS
Baking-Powder, 38
Low-Fat Buttermilk, 39
Black-Eyed Peas, 133

BLUEBERRIES
Cheesecake, 59
Very Berry Muffins, 44
Blueberry Cheesecake, 59
Blue-Ribbon Brownie Trifle, 78
Blue-Ribbon Brownies, 78
Blue-Ribbon Cornbread, 45

Blue-Ribbon Frozen Snicker Dessert, 68
Blue-Ribbon Vegetables, 133

BRAN
Chocolate Muffins, 41
Bread-Pudding Breakfast Dish, 171

BREADS
1-2-3 Easy Rolls, 38
Apple-Carrot Muffins, 40
Apple-Raisin Muffins, 40
Baking-Powder Biscuits, 38
Banana Bread, 45
Banana Muffins, 41
Blue-Ribbon Cornbread, 45
Breakfast Bars, 46
Buttermilk Cornbread, 46
Carrot Patties, 47
Chewy Fruit-and-Oatmeal Bars, 47
Chocolate Bran Muffins, 41
Easy Rolls, 39
French Toast, 48
Fresh Cranberry Muffins, 42
Garlic-Mustard Bread, 49
Honey Whole-Wheat Bread, 49
Light Waffles, 50
Low-Fat Buttermilk Biscuits, 39
Oatmeal-Apple Pancakes, 50
Orange Blossom Muffins, 42
Orange Rolls, 39
Sausage and Cheese Muffins, 43
Spinach Bread, 51
Tropical Muffins, 43
Very Berry Blueberry Muffins, 44
Breakfast Bars, 46

BROCCOLI

Cauliflower Salad, 144
Lasagna Rolls, 104
Salad, 143
Broccoli and Cauliflower Salad, 144
Broccoli Lasagna Rolls, 104
Broccoli Salad, 143
Brown Rice Jambalaya, 112

BROWNIES

Blue-Ribbon, 78
Blue-Ribbon Trifle, 78
Brunswick Crock-Pot Stew, 122

BURRITOS

Tuna, 102
Venison, 98

BUTTERMILK

Cornbread, 46
Low-Fat Biscuits, 39
Buttermilk Cornbread, 46
Butternut Squash Soup, 156

CABBAGE

Jambalaya, 87
Rolls, 134
Cabbage Jambalaya, 87
Cabbage Rolls, 134
Cajun Meat Loaf, 87

CAKES

Peach Pudding, 64
Sugar-Free Applesauce, 66
Cappuccino Mix, 55
Caramel Apple Salad, 144
Carrot Patties, 47

CARROTS

Apple Muffins, 40
Cauliflower and, 134
Lemon and Basil, 136
Orange-Glazed, 138
Patties, 47
Pineapple, 139

CASSEROLES

Chicken, 115
Creamy Corn, 134
Italian Vegetarian, 135
Shrimp, 102
Squash, 142
Sweet Potato and Apple, 142
Taco Chicken, 129
Turkey-Sausage and Spaghetti, 130
Zucchini, 142

CAULIFLOWER

Broccoli Salad, 144
and Carrots, 134
Cauliflower and Carrots, 134
Cheddar Cheese Soup, 157

CHEESE

Dip, 165
Enchiladas, 103
Macaroni, 136
Pineapple Ball, 33
Sausage Muffins, 43
Soup, 157
Spinach Manicotti, 107
Cheese Dip, 165
Cheese Enchiladas, 103

CHEESECAKES

Blueberry, 59
Chocolate and Peanut Butter Pie, 59
Fruit Delight, 61
Lemon-Cherry, 63
Mini, 63
White-Chocolate, 67

CHERRY

Lemon Cheesecake, 63
Chewy Fruit-and-Oatmeal Bars, 47

CHICKEN

Balsamic with Rosemary, 111
Barbecue Kabobs, 111
Casserole, 115
Chili Nachos, 119
Crock-Pot, 119
Curry, 115
Cyndi's Waterford Lakes, 120
Double T Mexican, 120
and Dumplings, 113
Easy Fajita Wraps, 121
Easy Oven-Baked, 122
Easy Spaghetti, 121
in Foil, 116
Garlic Fillets in Balsamic Vinegar, 122
Gilmer's Best Potpie, 123
Gilmont with Alfredo Sauce, 123
Mega Vegetable Soup, 158
Mexican, 124
Oven-Fried, 124
Parmesan Italiano, 116
and Pasta, 113
Pasta Toss, 116
Ranch-Style Breaded, 125

Reuben Bake, 117
and Rice, 114
and Rice Potpie, 114
Salad, 117
Sandy's Potpie, 125
Sesame Baked, 126
Slow "Souper" Chile, 126
Slow-Cooked Orange, 127
Smothered Italian, 127
Spaghetti, 117
Speedy Soup, 160
Spinach Salad, 145
Stuffed Breasts, 128
Stuffed Manicotti, 118
Supreme, 118
Sweet-and-Sour, 128
Taco Casserole, 129
Chicken and Dumplings, 113
Chicken and Pasta, 113
Chicken and Rice, 114
Chicken and Rice Potpie, 114
Chicken Casserole, 114
Chicken Curry, 115
Chicken in Foil, 115
Chicken Parmesan Italiano, 116
Chicken Pasta Toss, 116
Chicken Reuben Bake, 116
Chicken Salad, 117
Chicken Spaghetti, 117
Chicken Supreme, 118
Chicken-Stuffed Manicotti, 118

CHILI
Chicken Nachos, 119
Superb, 96

Chili-Chicken Nachos, 119
Chinese Coleslaw, 145

CHOCOLATE
Banana Cream Pie, 60
Bran Muffins, 41
Eclair Dessert, 79
Fruit Dip, 166
Homemade Ice Cream, 69
Ice Cream, 68
Mint Pie, 60
Mocha Mousse, 73
and Peanut Butter
  Cheesecake Pie, 59
Chocolate Banana Cream Pie, 60
Chocolate Banana Muffins, 41
Chocolate Eclair Dessert, 79
Chocolate Ice Cream, 68
Chocolate Mint Pie, 60
Chocolate Mocha Mousse, 73
White Cheesecake, 67

COBBLER
Apple, 76

COCONUT
Pineapple Pie, 65

COLESLAW
Chinese, 145
Southern Belle, 152
Confetti Party Salad, 146
Cool Lime Gelatin, 72

CORN
Creamy Casserole, 134

CORNBREAD
Blue-Ribbon, 45

Buttermilk, 46
Dressing, 48
Gravy for Dressing, 168
Salad, 47
Cornbread Dressing, 48
Cornbread Salad, 147
Cottage Salad, 147

CRANBERRIES
Light Mousse, 74
Muffins, 42
Punch, 55
Quick Punch, 56
Cranberry Punch, 55
Creamy Corn Casserole, 134
Creamy Fruit Salad, 148
Creamy Pumpkin Soufflé, 61

CRISP
Apple, 76
Fruit, 80
Crispy Zucchini Coins, 135

CROCK-POT
Aunt Lottie's Enchiladas, 86
Brunswick Stew, 112
Chicken, 119
Crock-Pot Chicken, 119

CUCUMBER
Best Friend's Dip, 165

CURRY
Chicken Curry, 115
Cyndi's Waterford Lakes Chicken,
  120

DESSERTS AND SWEETS
Apple Cobbler, 76

Apple Crisp, 76
Apple Dessert, 77
Apple Salad Mold, 71
Baked Apples, 77
Banana-Berry Cream Pie, 58
Banana-Split Dessert, 77
Blueberry Cheesecake, 59
Blue-Ribbon Brownie Trifle, 78
Blue-Ribbon Brownies, 78
Blue-Ribbon Frozen Snicker
    Dessert, 68
Chocolate and Peanut Butter
    Cheesecake Pie, 59
Chocolate Banana Cream Pie, 60
Chocolate Eclair Dessert, 79
Chocolate Ice Cream, 68
Chocolate Mint Pie, 60
Chocolate-Mocha Mousse, 73
Cool Lime Gelatin, 72
Creamy Pumpkin Soufflé, 61
First Place Banana Pudding, 73
Fluffy Fruit Dessert, 79
Frozen Pineapple-Banana Cups, 69
Fruit Crisp, 80
Fruit Delight Cheesecake, 61
Fruit Fluff, 72
Fruit Salad, 80
Homemade Chocolate Ice Cream,
    69
Key Lime Pie, 62
Lemon Icebox Dessert, 70
Lemon-Cherry Cheesecake, 63
Light and Easy No-Crust Pumpkin
    Pie, 74

Light and Luscious Orange Bars, 70
Light Cranberry Mousse, 74
Minicheesecakes, 63
Oatmeal Delight, 81
Oatmeal-Pecan Bars, 81
Peach Pudding Cake, 64
Pie-Pan Apple Tart, 64
Pineapple Dream, 82
Pineapple-Coconut Pie, 65
Rich and Creamy Banana Pudding,
    75
Strawberry Surprise, 82
Strawberry Trifle, 65
Sugar-Free Apple Pie, 66
Sugar-Free Applesauce Cake, 66
Sugar-Free Strawberry Pie, 67
Three-Layer Apple-Raisin Pie, 67
Tropical Pudding, 75
White-Chocolate Cheesecake, 67
Yogurt Soft-Serve Surprise, 83

DIPS
    Best Friend's Cucumber, 165
    Cheese, 165
    Chocolate Fruit, 166
    Fruit, 166
    Pizza, 166
    Quick Bean, 167
    Shrimp, 167
    Spinach, 168
Double T Mexican Chicken, 120
DRESSINGS
    Cornbread, 48
    Fat-Free Italian, 170
    Gravy for Cornbread, 168

Raspberry Vinaigrette, 171
DUMPLINGS
    Chicken, 113
    Old-Fashioned Strip, 172
Easy Beef or Venison Stew, 88
Easy Chicken Fajita Wraps, 121
Easy Chicken Spaghetti, 121
Easy Oven-Baked Chicken, 122
Easy Rolls, 39
Easy Summer Salad, 148
ECLAIRS
    Chocolate Dessert, 79
EGGS
    No-Yolk Deviled, 32
    Healthy Greek Omlet, 105
ENCHILADAS
    Aunt Lottie's Crock-Pot, 86
    Cheese, 103
    Green, 104
Extraordinary Baked Salmon, 99
FAJITA
    Easy Chicken Wraps, 121
Fat-Free Italian Dressing, 170
First Place Banana Pudding, 73
FISH AND SEAFOOD
    Baked Stuffed Fish, 99
    Extraordinary Baked Salmon, 99
    Quick and Easy Shrimp Creole, 100
    Seafood Primavera, 101
    Shrimp Casserole, 102
    Tuna Burrito, 102
Fluffy Fruit Dessert, 79
French Bread Vegetable Pizza, 104

NEW FIRST PLACE FAVORITES

Index

French Toast, 48
Fresh Cranberry Muffins, 42
Fresh Garden Salad, 149
Frozen Pineapple-Banana Cups, 69

FRUIT
  Chewy Oatmeal Bars, 47
  Chocolate Dip, 166
  Creamy Salad, 148
  Crisp, 80
  Delight Cheesecake, 61
  Dip, 166
  Fluff, 72
  Fluffy Dessert, 79
  Golden Ham, 110
  Salad, 80
Fruit Crisp, 80
Fruit Delight Cheesecake, 61
Fruit Dip, 166
Fruit Salad, 80

GARLIC
  Chicken Fillets in Balsamic Vinegar,
    122
  Mustard Bread, 49
  Hot Roasted Potatoes, 135
Garlic Chicken Fillets in Balsamic
    Vinegar, 122
Garlic-Mustard Bread, 49

GELATIN
  Cool Lime, 72
  Pineapple Salad, 151
Gilmer's Best Chicken Potpie, 123
Gilmont Chicken with Alfredo Sauce,
    123
Golden Fruited Ham. 110

Grape Salad, 149
Gravy for Cornbread Dressing, 168

GREEK
  Healthy Omelet, 105
  Spaghetti, 105
Greek Spaghetti, 105
Green Enchiladas, 104
Green-Pepper Steak, 89

HAM
  Golden Fruited, 110
Healthy Greek Omelet, 105
Homemade Chocolate Ice Cream, 69
Honey Whole-Wheat Bread, 49
Hot Garlic-Roasted Potatoes, 135

ICE CREAM
  Chocolate, 68
  Homemade Chocolate, 69

ITALIAN
  Chicken Parmesan, 116
  Fat-Free Dressing, 170
  Garden Soup, 157
  Marinated Green Beans, 149
  Smothered Chicken, 127
  Vegetarian Casserole, 135
  Zucchini Sauté, 136
Italian Garden Soup, 157
Italian Vegetarian Casserole, 135
Italian Zucchini Sauté, 136

JAMBALAYA
  Brown Rice, 112
  Cabbage, 87
Jamie's Mexican Lasagna, 90

KABOBS
  Barbecue Chicken, 111
Key Lime Pie, 62

LASAGNA
  Broccoli Rolls, 104
  Jamie's Mexican, 90
  Spinach, 108
  Stay-Slim, 95

LATTE
  Anytime Chocolate, 54
Lemon and Basil Carrots, 136
Lemon Icebox Dessert, 70
Lemon-Cherry Cheesecake, 163

LEMONS
  Basil Carrots, 136
  Cherry Cheesecake, 63
  Icebox Dessert, 70
  Soy Basting Sauce, 170
Light and Easy No-Crust
    Pumpkin Pie, 74
Light and Luscious Orange Bars, 70
Light Cranberry Mousse, 74
Light Mexican Manicotti, 91
Light Waffles, 50

LIMES
  Cool Gelatin, 72
  Pie, 62
Linguine with Fresh Tomato Sauce,
    106

LO MEIN
  Pork, 110
Low-Fat Buttermilk Biscuits, 39
Macaroni and Cheese, 136

NEW FIRST PLACE FAVORITES

MALT

Quick and Easy Vanilla, 56
Marinated Italian Green Beans, 149
Marinated Vegetables, 150

MEAT LOAF

Cajun, 87

MEATBALLS

Swedish Meatballs, 96
Mega-Chicken Vegetable Soup, 158

MEXICAN

Chicken, 124
Double T Chicken, 120
Jamie's Lasagna, 90
Light Manicotti, 91
Venison Torte, 92
Mexican Chicken, 124
Mexican-Style Venison Torte, 92
Minicheesecakes, 63

MINT

Chocolate Pie, 60

MOCHA

Chocolate Mousse, 73

MOUSSE

Chocolate-Mocha, 73
Light Cranberry, 74

MUFFINS

Apple-Carrot, 40
Apple-Raisin, 40
Banana, 41
Chocolate Bran, 41
Fresh Cranberry, 42
Orange Blossom, 42

Sausage and Cheese, 43
Tropical, 43
Very Berry Blueberry, 44

NACHOS

Chili-Chicken, 119
No-Yolk Deviled Eggs, 32
Not-So-Sweet Potatoes, 137

OATMEAL

Apple Pancakes, 50
Chewy Fruit Bars, 47
Delight, 81
Pecan Bars, 81
Oatmeal Delight, 81
Oatmeal-Apple Pancakes, 50
Oatmeal-Pecan Bars, 81

OKRA

Succotash, 137
and Tomatoes, 137
Okra and Tomatoes, 137
Okra Succotash, 137
Old-Fashioned Strip Dumplings, 172

OMELET

Healthy Greek, 105
Orange Blossom Muffins, 42
Orange Rolls, 39
Orange-Glazed Carrots, 138

ORANGES

Blossom Muffins, 42
Glazed Carrots, 138
Light and Luscious Bars, 70
Pineapple Salad, 151
Rolls, 39
Slow-Cooked Chicken, 127

Oven-Fried Chicken, 124
Oven-Fried Green Tomatoes or
  Squash, 138
Oven-Fried Potatoes, 138

PANCAKES

Oatmeal-Apple, 50
Quick Potato, 140

PARMESAN

Chicken Italiano, 116
Party Sandwich, 33

PASTA

Chicken, 113
Chicken Spaghetti, 117
Chicken Toss, 116
Chicken-Stuffed Manicotti, 118
e Fagioli, 158
Easy Chicken Spaghetti, 121
Greek Spaghetti, 105
Light Mexican Manicotti, 91
Linguine with Fresh Tomato Sauce,
  106
Roasted Red Pepper, 107
Salad, 150
Sauce, 169
Spaghetti Deluxe, 93
Spinach and Cheese Manicotti, 107
Stuffed Shells, 109
Turkey-Sausage and Spaghetti
Casserole, 130
Vegetable Pesto Fettuccine, 109
Whole-Wheat Spiral Salad, 154
Pasta e Fagioli, 158
Pasta Salad, 150
Pasta Sauce, 169

Peach Pudding Cake, 64

PEANUT BUTTER
Chocolate Cheesecake Pie, 59
Pearl's Tuna Salad, 151

PEAS
and Asparagus, 139
Black-Eyed, 133
Peppered Sugar Snap, 139
Peas and Asparagus, 139

PECAN
Oatmeal-Pecan Bars, 81
Peppered Sugar-Snap Peas, 139
Pie-Pan Apple Tart, 64

PIES
Banana-Berry Cream, 58
Chocolate and Peanut Butter
Cheesecake, 59
Chocolate Banana Cream, 60
Chocolate Mint, 60
Key Lime, 62
Light and Easy No-Crust
Pumpkin, 74
Pie-Pan Apple Tart, 64
Pineapple-Coconut, 65
Shepherd's, 93
Sugar-Free Apple, 66
Sugar-Free Strawberry, 67
Tamale, 97
Three-Layer Apple-Raisin, 67

PINEAPPLE
Carrots, 139
Cheese Ball, 33
Coconut Pie, 65

Dream, 82
Frozen Banana Cups, 69
Gelatin Salad, 151
Orange Salad, 152
Pineapple Carrots, 139
Pineapple Cheese Ball, 33
Pineapple Dream, 82
Pineapple Gelatin Salad, 151
Pineapple-Coconut Pie, 65
Pineapple-Orange Salad, 152
Pinto Beans á la Juan, 140
Pita Pizza, 106

PIZZA
Dip, 166
French Bread Vegetable, 104
Pita, 106
Sauce, 169
Pizza Dip, 166
Pizza Sauce, 169

PORK
Golden Fruited Ham, 110
Lo Mein, 110
Pork Lo Mein, 110

POTATOES
Apple Casserole, 142
Hot Garlic-Roasted, 135
Not-So-Sweet, 137
Quick Pancakes, 140
Savory Soup, 159
Smoked-Sausage Soup, 159
Southwest-Style Salad, 153
Spicy Sweet, 141

POTPIE
Chicken and Rice, 114
Gilmer's Best Chicken, 123
Sandy's Chicken, 125

POULTRY
Balsamic Chicken with Rosemary, 111
Barbecue Chicken Kabobs, 111
Brown Rice Jambalaya, 112
Brunswick Crock-Pot Stew, 112
Chicken and Dumplings, 113
Chicken and Pasta, 113
Chicken and Rice, 114
Chicken and Rice Potpie, 114
Chicken Casserole, 115
Chicken Curry, 115
Chicken in Foil, 116
Chicken Parmesan Italiano, 116
Chicken Pasta Toss, 116
Chicken Reuben Bake, 117
Chicken Salad, 117
Chicken Spaghetti, 117
Chicken Supreme, 118
Chicken-Stuffed Manicotti, 118
Chili-Chicken Nachos, 119
Crock-Pot Chicken, 119
Cyndi's Waterford Lakes Chicken,
120
Double T Mexican Chicken, 120
Easy Chicken Fajita Wraps, 121
Easy Chicken Spaghetti, 121
Easy Oven-Baked Chicken, 122
Garlic Chicken Fillets in Balsamic
Vinegar, 122
Gilmer's Best Chicken Potpie, 123

Gilmont Chicken with Alfredo Sauce, 123
Mexican Chicken, 124
Oven-Fried Chicken, 124
Ranch-Style Breaded Chicken, 125
Sandy's Chicken Potpie, 125
Sesame Baked Chicken, 126
Slow "Souper" Chile-Chicken, 126
Slow-Cooked Orange Chicken, 127
Smothered Italian Chicken, 127
Stuffed Chicken Breasts, 128
Sweet-and-Sour Chicken, 128
Taco Chicken Casserole, 129
Turkey Barbecue, 129
Turkey-Sausage and Spaghetti
    Casserole, 130

PRIMAVERA
    Seafood, 101

PUDDINGS
    Bread Breakfast Dish, 171
    First Place Banana, 73
    Peach Cake, 64
    Rich and Creamy Banana, 75
    Tropical, 75

PUMPKIN
    Creamy Soufflé, 61
    Light and Easy No-Crust Pie, 74

PUNCH
    Cranberry, 55
    Quick Cranberry, 56

QUESADILLAS
    Vegetarian, 35
Quick and Easy Shrimp Creole, 100

Quick and Easy Vanilla Malt, 56
Quick Cranberry Punch, 56
Quick Potato Pancakes, 140

RAISINS
    Apple Muffins, 40
    Three-Layer Apple Pie, 67
Ranch-Style Breaded Chicken, 125
Raspberry Vinaigrette Dressing, 171

REUBEN
    Chicken Bake, 116

RICE
    Brown Jambalaya, 112
    Chicken, 114
    Chicken Potpie, 114
Rich and Creamy Banana Pudding, 75
Roasted Red Pepper Pasta, 107

ROLLS
    1-2-3 Easy, 38
    Broccoli Lasagna, 104
    Cabbage, 134
    Easy, 39
    Orange, 39
    Tortilla Roll-Ups, 34

SALADS
    Apple Mold, 71
    Beet, 143
    Broccoli, 143
    Broccoli-Cauliflower, 144
    Caramel Apple, 144
    Chicken, 117
    Chicken-Spinach, 145
    Confetti Party, 146
    Cornbread, 147

Cottage, 147
Creamy Fruit, 148
Easy Summer, 148
Fresh Garden, 149
Fruit, 80
Grape, 149
Pasta, 150
Pearl's Tuna, 151
Pineapple Gelatin, 151
Pineapple-Orange, 152
Southwest-Style Potato, 153
Spinach, 153
Waldorf, 154
Whole-Wheat Spirals, 154

SALMON
    Extraordinary Baked, 99

SANDWICHES
Party, 33
Sandy's Chicken Potpie, 125

SAUCES
    Gilmont Chicken with Alfredo, 123
    Linguine with Fresh Tomato, 106
    Pasta, 169
    Pizza, 169
    Soy-Lemon Basting, 170

SAUSAGE
    Cheese Muffins, 43
    Potato Soup, 159
    Spaghetti Casserole, 130
Sausage and Cheese Muffins, 43
Savory Potato Soup, 159
Seafood Primavera, 101
Sesame Baked Chicken, 126

SHAKE
   Banana Milk Shake, 54
Shepherd's Pie, 93

SHRIMP
   Casserole, 102
   Dip, 167
   Quick and Easy Creole, 100
Shrimp Casserole, 102
Shrimp Dip, 167

SIDE DISHES
   Baked Tomatoes, 132
   Black-Eyed Peas, 133
   Blue-Ribbon Vegetables, 133
   Cabbage Rolls, 134
   Cauliflower and Carrots, 134
   Creamy Corn Casserole, 134
   Crispy Zucchini Coins, 135
   Hot Garlic-Roasted Potatoes, 135
   Italian Vegetarian Casserole, 135
   Italian Zucchini Sauté, 136
   Lemon and Basil Carrots, 136
   Macaroni and Cheese, 136
   Not-So-Sweet Potatoes, 137
   Okra and Tomatoes, 137
   Okra Succotash, 137
   Orange-Glazed Carrots, 138
   Oven-Fried Green Tomatoes or
      Squash, 138
   Oven-Fried Potatoes, 138
   Peas and Asparagus, 139
   Peppered Sugar-Snap Peas, 139
   Pineapple Carrots, 139
   Pinto Beans á la Juan, 140
   Quick Potato Pancakes, 140

Spicy Sweet Potatoes, 141
Squash Bake, 141
Squash Casserole, 142
Sweet Potato and Apple Casserole,
   142
Zucchini Casserole, 142
Simple Veggie Tortillas, 34
Slow "Souper" Chile-Chicken, 126
Slow-Cooked Orange Chicken, 127
Smoked-Sausage and Potato Soup,
   159

SMOOTHIES
   Banana-Berry, 55
   Strawberry, 56
   Tutti-Frutti, 57
Smothered Italian Chicken, 127

SOUFFLÉS
   Creamy Pumpkin, 61

SOUPS
   Butternut Squash, 156
   Cheddar Cheese, 157
   Italian Garden, 157
   Pasta e Fagioli, 158
   Mega-Chicken Vegetable, 158
   Savory Potato, 159
   Smoked-Sausage and Potato, 159
   Speedy Chicken, 160
   Taco, 160
   White Bean, 161
Southern Belle Coleslaw, 152
Southwest-Style Potato Salad, 153
Soy-Lemon Basting Sauce, 170
Spaghetti Deluxe, 93
Speedy Chicken Soup, 160

Spicy Sweet Potatoes, 141
Spicy Swiss Steak, 94

SPINACH
   Artichoke Spread, 167
   Bread, 51
   Cheese Manicotti, 107
   Chicken-Salad, 145
   Dip, 168
   Lasagna, 108
   Salad, 153
   Wraps, 34
Spinach and Artichoke Spread, 167
Spinach and Cheese Manicotti, 107
Spinach Bread, 51
Spinach Dip, 168
Spinach Lasagna, 108
Spinach Salad, 153
Spinach Wraps, 34
Spoonburgers Barbecue, 94

SPREADS
   Apricot, 164
   Spinach and Artichoke, 167

SQUASH
   Bake, 141
   Butternut Soup, 156
   Casserole, 142
   Oven-Fried, 138
Squash Bake, 141
Squash Casserole, 142
Stay-Slim Lasagna, 95

STEWS
   Brunswick Crock-Pot, 112
   Easy Beef or Venison, 88

STRAWBERRIES
   Smoothie, 56
   Sugar-Free Pie, 67
   Surprise, 82
   Trifle, 65
Strawberry Smoothie, 56
Strawberry Surprise, 82
Strawberry Trifle, 65
Stuffed Chicken Breasts, 128
Stuffed Pasta Shells, 109

SUCCOTASH
   Okra, 137
Sugar-Free Apple Pie, 66
Sugar-Free Applesauce Cake, 66
Sugar-Free Strawberry Pie, 67
Superb Chili and Beans, 96
Swedish Meatballs, 96
Sweet Potato and Apple Casserole, 142
Sweet-and-Sour Chicken, 128

SWISS
   Spicy Swiss Steak, 94
Taco Chicken Casserole, 129
Taco Soup, 160
Tamale Pie, 97

TARTS
   Pie-Pan Apple, 64
Teague Tortilla Bake, 98
Three-Layer Apple-Raisin Pie, 67

TOAST
   French, 48

TOMATOES
   Baked, 132
   Linguine with Fresh Sauce, 137

Okra, 137
Oven-Fried, 138

TORTE
   Mexican-Style Venison, 92
Tortilla Roll-Ups, 34

TORTILLAS
   Roll-Ups, 34
   Simple Veggie, 34
   Teague Bake, 98

TRIFLE
   Blue-Ribbon Brownie, 78
   Strawberry, 65
Tropical Muffins, 43
Tropical Pudding, 75

TUNA
   Burrito, 102
   Pearl's Salad, 151
Tuna Burrito, 102

TURKEY
   Barbecue, 129
   Sausage and Spaghetti Casserole, 130
Turkey Barbecue, 129
Turkey-Sausage and Spaghetti Casserole, 130
Tutti-Frutti Smoothie, 57
Vegetable Pesto Fettucine, 109

VEGETABLES
   Blue-Ribbon, 133
   French Bread Pizza, 104
   Italian Casserole, 135
   Marinated, 150
   Mega-Chicken Soup, 158

Pesto Fettucine, 109
Quesadillas, 35
Simple Tortillas, 34
Vegetarian Quesadillas, 35

VENISON
   Burritos, 98
   Easy Stew, 88
   Mexican-Style Torte, 92
Venison Burritos, 98
Very Berry Blueberry Muffins, 44

WAFFLES
   Light, 50
Waldorf Salad, 154
Wassail, 57
White Bean Soup, 161
White-Chocolate Cheesecake, 67
Whole-Wheat Spirals Salad, 154

WRAPS
   Easy Chicken Fajita, 121
   Spinach, 34
Yogurt Soft-Serve Surprise, 83

ZUCCHINI
   Casserole, 142
   Crispy Coins, 135
   Italian Sauté, 136
Zucchini Casserole, 142

THE BIBLE'S WAY TO WEIGHT LOSS

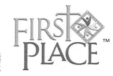

**The Bible-Based Weight-Loss Program
Used by Over a Half Million People!**

Are you one of the millions of disheartened dieters who've tried one fad diet after another without success? If so, your search for a successful diet is over! First Place is the proven weight-loss program, born over 20 years ago in the First Baptist Church of Houston.

But First Place does much more than help you take off weight and keep it off. This Bible-based program will transform your life in every way—physically, mentally, spiritually and emotionally. Now's the time to join!

ESSENTIAL FIRST PLACE PROGRAM MATERIALS

Group Leaders Need:

■ **Group Starter Kit**
ISBN 08307.28708

This kit has everything group leaders need to help others change their lives forever by giving Christ first place!

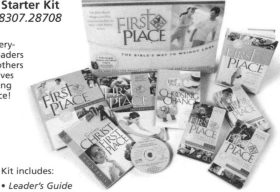

Kit includes:
• *Leader's Guide*
• *Member's Guide*
• *Giving Christ First Place Bible Study*
  with Scripture Memory Music CD
• *Choosing to Change* by Carole Lewis
• *First Place* by Carole Lewis with Terry Whalin
• *Orientation* Video
• *Nine Commitments* Video
• *Food Exchange Plan* Video
• *An Introduction to First Place* Video

Group Members Need:

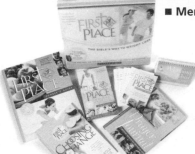

■ **Member's Kit** • *ISBN 08307.28694*

All the material is easy to understand and spells out principles members can easily apply in their daily lives.

Kit includes:

• *Member's Guide*
• *Choosing to Change* by Carole Lewis
• 13 Commitment Records
• Four Motivational Audiocassettes
• *Prayer Journal*
• *Walking in the Word:*
  Scripture Memory Verses

■ **First Place Bible Study**

**Giving Christ
First Place
Bible Study**
with Scripture
Memory Music CD

Bible Study
ISBN 08307.28643

Many other First Place Bible studies are available. Visit www.firstplace.org for a complete listing

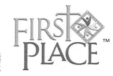

044267

Available at your local Christian bookstore or by calling **1-800-4-GOSPEL**.
Join the First Place community at www.firstplace.org

Gospel Light

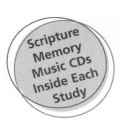
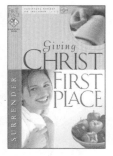
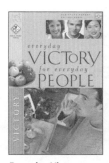
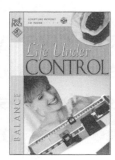
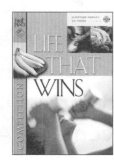
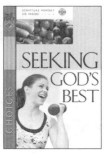
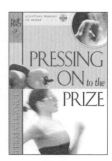
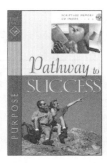
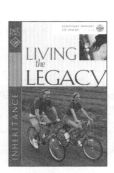
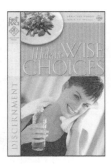
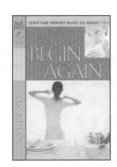
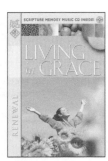
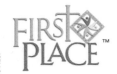

Inspiration & Information Everymonth
Subscribe Today!

Every newsletter gives you:

- New recipes
- Food tips
- Coming events
- Helpful articles
- Inspiring testimonies
- And much more!

Register for our FREE e-newsletter at www.firstplace.org

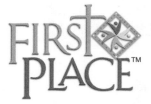

FIRST PLACE™

A Must-Have Publication for all First Place Leaders & Members!

To receive information about special events & products

Stay in the Loop!
Register Your Group!

Visit us online at
www.firstplace.org
or return the form to the right

044267

Biblically Based Reading
for Healthy Living

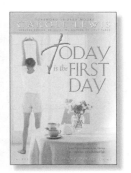

**Today Is
the First Day**

Daily Encouragement on
the Journey to Weight
Loss and a Balanced Life
Carole Lewis,
General Editor
Hardcover
ISBN 08307.30656

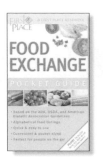

**First Place
Food Exchange
Pocket Guide**

Convenient pocket-sized
listing of all First Place
food exchanges and fast
food favorites.
Mass
ISBN 08307.32322

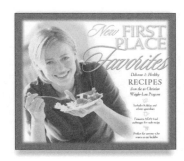

**New First Place
Favorites**

Favorite Recipes
from the Nation's
leading Christian
Weight-Loss Program
Hardcover
ISBN 08307.32314

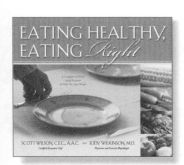

**Eating Healthy,
Eating Right**

A Complete 16-Week
Meal Planner to Help You
Lose Weight
Scott Wilson,
C.I.C., A.A.C.
and *Jody Wilkinson*, M.D.
Hardcover
ISBN 08307.30222

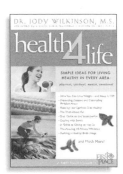

Health 4 Life

55 Simple Ideas
for Living Healthy in
Every Area
Jody Wilkinson, M.D.
Paperback
ISBN 08307.30516

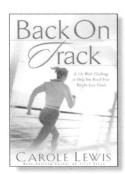

Back on Track

A 16-Week Challenge
to Help You Reach Your
Weight-Loss Goals
Carole Lewis
Paperback
ISBN 08307.32586

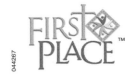

044267

Available at your local Christian bookstore or by calling **1-800-4-GOSPEL**.
Join the First Place community at www.firstplace.org

Gospel Light